CANNABIS FOR CREATIVES

How 32 Artists Enhance and Sustain Inspiration

JORDANA WRIGHT

Cannabis for Creatives
Jordana Wright

ISBN: 978-1-68198-695-1
1st Edition (1st printing, January 2022)
© 2022 Jordana Wright
Additional image credits on page 229

Rocky Nook Inc.
1010 B Street, Suite 350
San Rafael, CA 94901
USA

www.rockynook.com

Distributed in the UK and Europe by Publishers Group UK
Distributed in the U.S. and all other territories by Ingram Publisher Services

Library of Congress Control Number: 2021937330

Editor: Jocelyn Howell
Project manager: Lisa Brazieal
Marketing coordinator: Mercedes Murray
Interior design: Jake Flaherty
Layout and type: Danielle Foster
Cover art and design: Nelson Ruger

This book is printed on acid-free paper.
Printed in Korea

CONTENTS

PREFACE   vii

Introduction
UNCOVERING THE RELATIONSHIP BETWEEN
CREATIVITY AND CANNABIS   1

Chapter 1
CANNABIS USE THROUGH HISTORY   9

Chapter 2
STUDYING CREATIVITY   21

Chapter 3
CANNABIS AND THE BRAIN   39

Chapter 4
UNDERSTANDING THE PLANT   65

Chapter 5
CANNABIS AND CREATIVITY: THE INTERVIEWS   93

     Artist Profile: Juerg Federer   95
     Artist Interview: Ray Benson   100
     Artist Profile: Daniela Valdez   107
     Artist Profile: Michael Marras   112
     Artist Interview: Carlos Mandelaveitia   117
     Artist Profile: Christopher O'Riley   124
     Artist Interview: Garrett Shore   129
     Artist Profile: Anna Pollock   136
     Artist Interview: Nelson Ruger   142

Artist Profile: Nathaniel C. Hunter   149

Artist Interview: Kenton Williams   152

Artist Profile: Nikki Barber   157

Artist Profile: Dope Chief   164

Artist Interview: Barrett Guzaldo   169

Artist Profile: Kael Mendoza   175

Artist Interview: Mark Karan   180

Artist Profile: Colton Clifford   186

Artist Interview: Robert Poehler   191

Artist Profile: Mark McDowell   198

Artist Interview: Kay Villamin   203

Chapter 6

EXPLORING YOUR OWN CREATIVITY WITH CANNABIS   213

Conclusion

CONTINUING THE CYCLE OF CREATIVITY   223

GLOSSARY   227

TEXT REFERENCES AND IMAGE CITATIONS   229

ACKNOWLEDGMENTS   233

INDEX   235

PREFACE

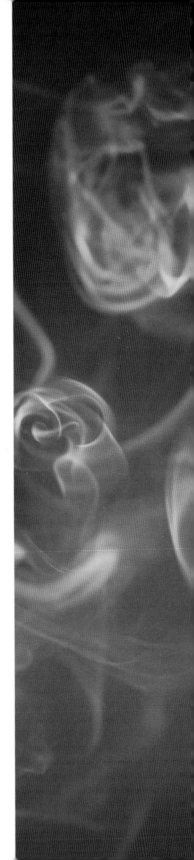

We are all born creative. When we're young and our concepts of the world are based on possibility rather than doubt, limitation, or worry, our imaginations carry us through wild and inventive scenarios. The worlds we can create in our minds are boundless, so we build block towers, imagining medieval cities, and we transform cardboard boxes into rocket ships.

Some of our earliest imaginings are based in the world we know, and we play to practice existing in that world. Other imaginings are pure creation. They're inspired by things we've experienced but unrestricted by the rules and realities of the world we will one day inhabit as adults. As we grow and learn to exist more in practical realities, imaginative play dwindles. We may still experience creative pursuits and explorations, but our focus shifts to the final product: a painting, a graded project for school, a recipe, etc. We stop creating for the act of creation itself and instead create for results. If no result occurs, what was the point?

I remember my early interactions with cannabis as a return to the imaginative state of my childhood. I was a teenager when I began experimenting with pot—not that far from childhood, but already feeling boundaries and hard edges where once only pure possibility existed. Most of my creative projects were either in art class at school or following along with a tutorial. Pure, self-guided creation was rarer and harder to come by.

My creative education in school was highly structured and focused more on teaching an existing language of art than it was about inspiring kids to invent and define their own words. Cannabis reawakened some of that free-flowing creativity in me. It reminded me that sometimes you must build things purely for the experience of building them and

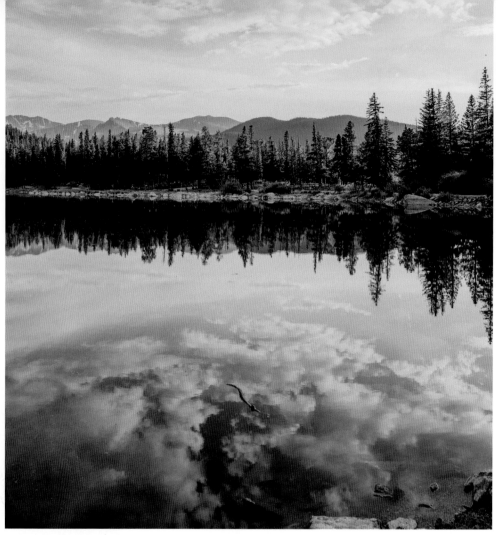

Colorado offers the perfect combination of legal cannabis and photographic opportunities.

seeing what happens. Creation isn't just about assembling a polished product and showing the world how clever or talented you are. You create for the joy, the frustration, and the challenge of the process.

I've always felt an overwhelming impulse to create, and after exploring a wide variety of artistic pursuits, I found that photography best allowed me to interpret and intuit the world. I've worked as a professional photographer since 2006, but my first real camera, and the fulfillment it brought, came into my life the same year that I discovered pot. For me, cannabis and photography have been linked intrinsically from the start. Much of the way I think about and choose to depict the world has been influenced by the experiences I've had while high.

As cannabis has become more mainstream, I, like many of my pot-loving peers, feel more confident in discussing its effects on my thought process and my creative flow. I've managed to shake some of the shame that the American education system and well-intentioned programs such as the Drug Abuse Resistance Education (D.A.R.E.) instilled so many years ago. The world is waking up to the benefits of cannabis. Much of the United States has legalized cannabis for adult use, so rather than sending coded text messages and blowing pot smoke through paper towel tubes stuffed with dryer sheets to mask the smell (this is called a **sploof** and was a common smoking accessory in high school and college), we can shop in stores for flavors we like and smoke in our homes or backyards without concern.

As the acceptance and influence of cannabis grows, so has a long list of related terms and titles. Between these two covers, you may come across new terms or alternate names for things you don't recognize. Words highlighted in bold are defined in the glossary, so if you find yourself needing a refresher on **dab rigs**, **spliffs**, or **volcanoes**, the explanations await you there.

What follows is an exploration of the human mind—the magic spark called *creativity* that lives at the intersection of inspiration and execution, and a plant that has been an influential catalyst since our earliest civilizations. Inspired to find other cannabis enthusiasts who work in creative fields, I interviewed artists from a wide range of backgrounds and specialties. I hoped to learn about the commonalities and nuances of the creative experience and to form actionable ideas on how to harness pot's creative energy most effectively.

The experience of writing this book and engaging with this impressive collection of artists has confirmed some of my beliefs about pot, triggered new ideas about creativity, and reinforced the notion that

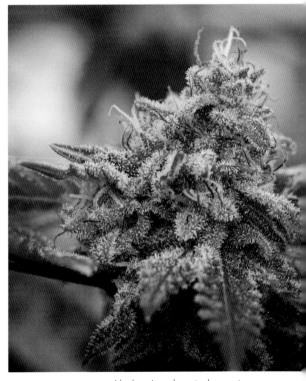

Alaskan Ice close to harvest

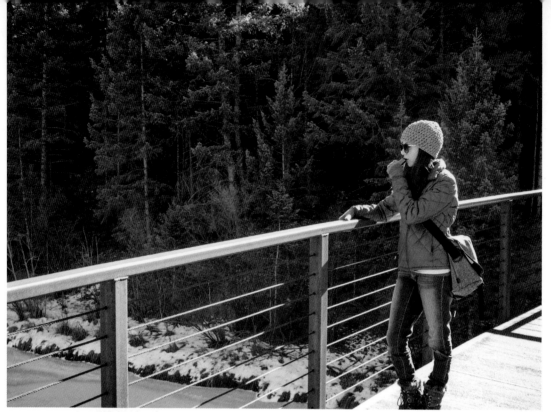

Enjoying a puff while out taking photos

something as magical as the act of artistic creation deserves at least a little experimentation with this mind-expanding and clarity-inducing super-plant we call cannabis, pot, weed, ganja, herb, chronic, and a variety of other names.

We're still early in the process of social and legal acceptance, so while it feels a little uncomfortable to put these words to paper, I believe so completely that cannabis has enriched my creative life that I want to help lessen the stigma and remind anyone who's reading this book that we are put on this earth to do more than create things for accolades or because someone told us to be productive.

If cannabis can help you rekindle that spark of imagination to explore and enjoy the inner workings of your mind and the world around you, then it just might be the most precious creative resource you will ever find. Whether you're a chef, a painter, or a person with plenty of creative energy with no idea where to start, thank you for joining me on this adventure and for being open to exploring your own creative journeys with cannabis.

UNCOVERING THE RELATIONSHIP BETWEEN CREATIVITY AND CANNABIS

What comes to your mind when you hear the word *creativity*? Do you imagine Renaissance artists pushing the boundaries of realistic representation? Do you think of Baroque composers inventing intricate threads and themes that expanded our ideas of musical scope and capability? Does your mind jump to modern revolutionaries, designing and inventing innovative technologies? Or do you picture yourself: crafting, cooking, singing, dancing, drawing, or dreaming?

In his short story *Everything's Eventual*, Stephen King wrote: "'Creativity is like a hand at the end of your arm. But a hand has many fingers, doesn't it? Think of those fingers as abilities. A creative person may write, paint, sculpt, or think up math formulae; he or she might dance or sing or play a musical instrument. Those are the fingers, but creativity is the hand that gives them life.'"

There are days when I wake up and feel a distinct impulse to create. It feels like a particular hunger that can only be sated by busying my hands and mind in an act of making. For many of us, it's fair to take King's words one step further and say: creativity is the hand that gives *us* life. Through our creativity, we invent new worlds to inhabit, follow driving impulses, and find a level of satisfaction that simply isn't provided by any other means.

What Is Creativity?

Creativity is a famously difficult concept to define succinctly. In fact, it's so elusive and amorphous that in academia, creativity is often discussed as *Creativity* (big C) vs. *creativity* (little c). We collectively think of big-C Creativity as genius-level or innovative artistic pursuits. Painting, sculpture, music, dance, theatre, poetry, and photography—all these very artistic genres belong to Creativity (big C). More practical pursuits requiring creative thinking to navigate the world successfully belong to creativity (little c). General problem-solving tasks, such as planning your errands in an order that allows you to make fewer left turns or organizing a seating arrangement so feuding family members don't cause drama at your wedding—these still require creativity, even if they don't feel terribly creative in practice.

In his book, *Keep Going: 10 Ways to Stay Creative in Good Times and Bad*, artist and author Austin Kleon wrote, "Being creative is never an end; it is a means to something

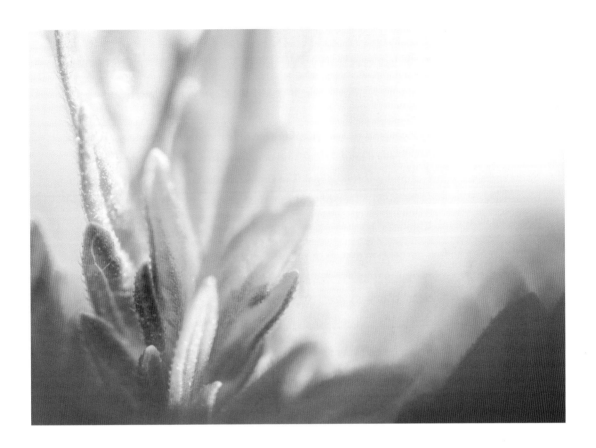

else. Creativity is just a tool. Creativity can be used to organize your living room, paint a masterpiece, or design a weapon of mass destruction." Creativity and creativity inhabit countless tasks and pursuits that we perform throughout our lives. While Creativity is more likely to feed our souls, creativity helps us manage our lives effectively.

Scientifically, there are many similarities in how Creativity and creativity are examined and measured, but most of the existing research focuses on creativity because society values it for productivity. With creativity, we are more efficient workers and more resourceful business owners. Research lives and dies with funding, so unless a researcher can demonstrate a practical application of their proposed work, our questions about Creativity go unanswered. As a result, we know much less about Creativity than many artists and neuroscientists would like, and Creativity and creativity are lumped together, however disparate they might be.

What Do We Know About
Cannabis and Creativity?

As of this writing (August 2021), cannabis remains federally illegal in the United States. Nevertheless, many states have implemented broad adult-use legalization. Several more have legalized medicinal cannabis use, while others have decriminalized cannabis, stopping short of allowing it to be legally manufactured and acquired. To date, only a handful of US states remain in which cannabis is fully illegal. The United States is slowly but surely trending toward acceptance of cannabis. In fact, 68% of Americans responded that they supported broad legalization of cannabis in a 2020 Gallup Poll.

Frustratingly, a shift in perception and state legalization isn't enough to facilitate easier academic study. For many, the regulations surrounding cannabis research may come as a surprise, but federal illegality and inconsistent state-to-state regulations are responsible for a wide variety of complications that scientists navigate when performing research.

Supply barriers are one of the biggest complications. Under infinitely greater scrutiny than your average trial-and-error grab-bag dispensary customer, scientists must seek approval from the National Institute on Drug Abuse (NIDA) and other government agencies to obtain cannabis samples for research purposes. It's a lengthy, complicated, and seemingly arbitrary approval process that impedes progress.

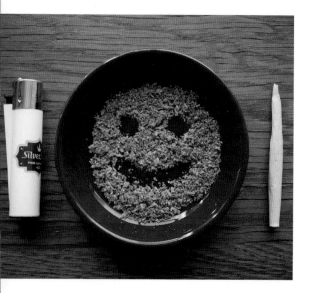

To make matters worse, until this year, all NIDA-approved studies had to obtain their cannabis samples from the official US cannabis farm at the University of Mississippi. Before you get too excited about the phrase "official US cannabis farm," you should know that they're hardly producing top-shelf buds. On the consumer market, high-Tetrahydrocannabinol (**THC**) percentage flower (18%–21% and beyond) is readily available and frequently relied upon for a variety of applications, medical and otherwise. Yet NIDA-approved samples are often reported to contain less than 10% THC. Scientists also complain about the quality and appearance of the samples they receive—a freeze dried, light green, ultra-fine powder. These samples are irrelevant compared to what consumers buy on the market, which results in heavily skewed data and less than reliable conclusions from studies.

Imagine that you've been smoking a 20% THC Gorilla Glue cannabis strain to help your back pain and insomnia. A **joint** in the evening does wonders. You enroll in a clinical study to help define the benefits of medical cannabis and receive a dose of NIDA-approved 5% THC pot. You can't just twist it up in a joint or smoke it in the **bong** like you do at home. Your cannabis dosage is administered as an intravenous injection. (Odd as it sounds, this is a common method in research for the sake of standardization.) Do you think that your body will respond as favorably toward the injected NIDA **ditch-weed** as the carefully bred commercial nuggets you're used to? Of course not, and the research data will skew toward pot being ineffective for pain and sleep.

Very recently, the DEA announced a new application process to expand the sources of cannabis for medical studies. It's a step forward, but like any new rollout, there have been complications, roadblocks, and

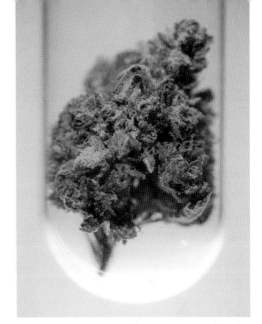

Bruce Banner is a strain that packs a punch with nearly 30% THC content!

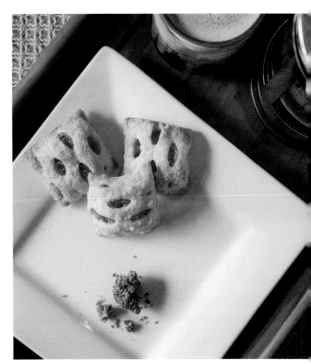

Once you find the right strain for your needs, habitual and reliable use increases effectiveness and quality of life.

bottlenecks that will take time to unravel. At best, we're still years away from broad, actionable conclusions that could make a difference in countless lives.

Biologists who aim to study cannabis purely as a specimen rather than as an administered **psychotropic** also have plenty of hoops to jump through. They're able to use samples of cannabis from sources all over the world, as long as they never bring any physical samples into government-owned or -funded laboratories, including state-funded universities and colleges. If you're a student at one of these universities, regulations like these will greatly diminish the work you can achieve in the pursuit of your education. These limitations add up, seriously obstructing official research channels in the conclusions that they can draw.

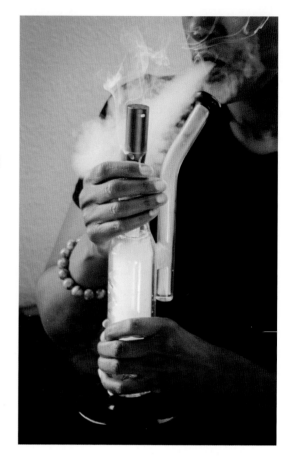

With so many limitations to navigate, very little research has been performed addressing the relationship between cannabis and creativity, and even fewer studies have been able to demonstrate a correlation between the two. Yet, we collectively know from the cultural zeitgeist that cannabis and creativity have been intertwined for a very, very long time.

Conversations About Cannabis and Creativity

When discussing cannabis use, laboratory science might be hindered, but social science excels. With an educational background in both anthropology and theatre, I believe that the most useful information isn't always found in data points and numbers, but in detailed accounts and storytelling. The words we choose to describe our experiences and the perspectives those experiences lead us to form are perhaps the simplest solution to understanding the relationship between cannabis and creativity.

As an anthropology student in a combined anthropology and sociology department, I used to struggle with the notion that data must be easily coded or quantified to draw effective conclusions. Sociology traffics in the quantitative, seeking statistically measurable patterns about populations for understanding human behavior. There's a lot of math in sociology, but formulas and data entry are not my preferred methods of analysis. My mind just doesn't work that way. Anthropology focuses on the qualitative in the study of culture. Interviews, case studies, and fieldwork best represent tangible traditions and group behavioral patterns. The anthropologist's approach values the individual insights to interpret the greater culture and community.

Anthropology taught me that when I had questions about cannabis and creativity inspired by my own experiences and pursuits, the best means of drawing conclusions was to ask the experts: those who use cannabis as part of their creative lives. Direct interviews promise a more complete understanding of the ways that cannabis and creativity relate than anything found in the results of a laboratory study. In speaking with this collection of artists, I learned about a wide array of unique and personal journeys to harness the psychoactive and medicinal effects of cannabis for the creation process. They vary wildly in a beautiful and surprising way. Humans may share physical structures and some behavioral commonalities, but a distinct individuality determines our creative processes and how we "get in the flow."

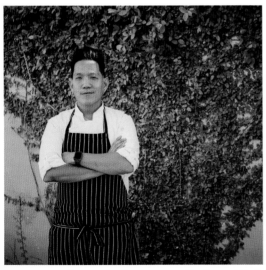 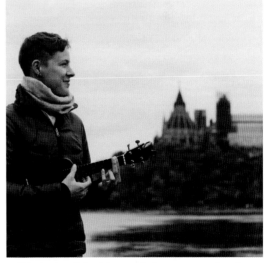

Interviews with cannabis-loving artists like Bruno Wu (left) and Trisha Smith (right) provided greater insights than statistics ever could.

Until we have a more precise means of studying these highly personal experiences, formulas and equations don't hold a candle to the conclusions we can draw through anecdotal accounts. With enough narrative evidence demonstrating a correlation between creativity and cannabis use, perhaps the need for greater study and new methods of analysis in the laboratory setting will be made abundantly clear.

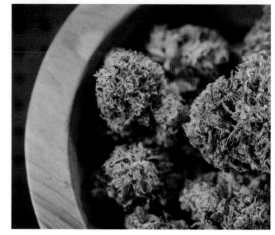

Citral Skunk

Exploring the Correlation

You don't have to perform interviews or delve into any intense research to know that cannabis and creativity are correlated in our collective consciousness. With so many artists over the years lauding the benefits of pot, we just *know* that weed speaks to our creative sides. Maybe you haven't given it any significant thought before, but with countless songs written about it, quotes from your favorite actors, and musings by successful CEOs, evidence has been mounting in the back of our minds to reinforce the connection.

In just a few minutes of searching online for "cannabis and creativity," you'll find a long and wide-ranging list of famous artists, musicians, authors, performers, and more who have used pot to get in the creative spirit. It's nothing new. We've been using cannabis for creative applications for generations. Even if you think you don't have cannabis as a touchstone in your cultural experience, it's there. If you've ever tapped your toes to the Beatles or the Rolling Stones, you've felt the indirect effects of cannabis.

Despite our collective notions, it's important to explore beyond the stereotype that weed makes you deep, insightful, and creative, just as we should look beyond the negative stereotypes of stoner laziness, fits of giggling ineptitude, and the PSA-promised loss of brain cells. Detailed conversations take our understanding of cannabis from the sphere of sound-bites and listicles to a nuanced explanation of how it's used, how it feels, why we like it, and what it can do for us.

CHAPTER 1

CANNABIS USE THROUGH HISTORY

It is nearly impossible to separate the human element from the history of cannabis. Humans have accepted the value of this plant for thousands of years, so with something as simple as a handful of seeds pocketed along a trade route, we've introduced it to nearly every continent on the planet and granted it access to some of the most defining eras in human history.

Practical, Medical, and Religious Use

Humanity's earliest cultures formed and developed through the religious and practical integration of plants. Whether seeking nourishment, medicine, or communication with the gods, plants represented a vital resource for all ancient cultures from the Maya to the nomadic tribes of Central Asia.

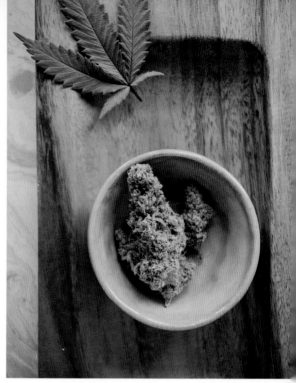

Medijuana

Some of the earliest evidence of cannabis use was found in China at the Pan-p'o village site. Dating back to 4,000 BCE, the site contained deposits of cannabis pollen and confirmed historians' beliefs that cannabis was a valued resource for ancient Chinese cultures. Not only was cannabis listed as a powerful medicine in the world's oldest pharmacopeia, but the Chinese relied on cannabis as a source of oil, grain, fiber, rope, and for an array of psychoactive uses. By around 1,000 BCE, cannabis was documented in India, where it was incorporated into medicine, the Hindu religion, and the search for psychoactive induced elation. For ancient cultures, cannabis was a plant that kept on giving.

In the centuries that followed, traders and explorers carried cannabis across mountain ranges and over oceans. It appeared in the Middle East by 430 BCE, where Scythians used it in funeral ceremonies. Similar to the modern tradition of **hotboxing**, they would burn large quantities of cannabis over a pyre and sit in an enclosed space with the smoke for its intoxicating effects.

CANNABIS FOR CREATIVES

Hemp, a non-psychoactive variety of cannabis, proliferated through the Mediterranean, Central and Northern Europe, and even reached Iceland thanks to the Vikings' appreciation for hemp's strength and durability when woven into rope. Cannabis's reach extended to the mountains of Tibet, was incorporated into birthing practices in Jerusalem, and was imported through Egypt to Ethiopia and beyond. Through European explorers, colonialism, and the slave trade, cannabis found its way to North, South, and Central America, where it was quickly adopted in cultural, medicinal, and agricultural practices.

In one form or another, cannabis traveled to every corner of the earth and found a home in countless cultures and civilizations. You could fill whole libraries with historical records of cannabis use for medicinal, religious, and spiritual purposes and still only scratch the surface.

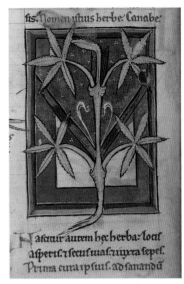

Cannabis was found in the pages of a 12th-century European pharmacopeia.

Cannabis's Artistic Applications Emerge

While ancient history primarily documented medical and religious uses of cannabis, modern history is teeming with examples of artistic communities exploring its creative capabilities. Artists separated by oceans, centuries, and the vast variability of the human experience are unified in the belief that pot brings inspiration to the forefront and fuels creation.

In exploring the history of cannabis and creativity, certain communities inevitably take center stage. Writers, with their command of descriptive language, impressive introspection, and ability to summarize complex concepts into relatable ideas, serve as invaluable interpreters of the cannabis experience. Musicians, with their ability to make audiences feel things through lyrics and melodies and their revered celebrity status, imbue the cannabis scene with glamour and swagger. Comedians and actors give voice to our inner monologues and capture the joy, hilarity, and, at times, intensity of the cannabis experience. Visual artists create food for the eyes, filling canvases with colorful symphonies that capture our attention and elevate our understanding of beauty and representation.

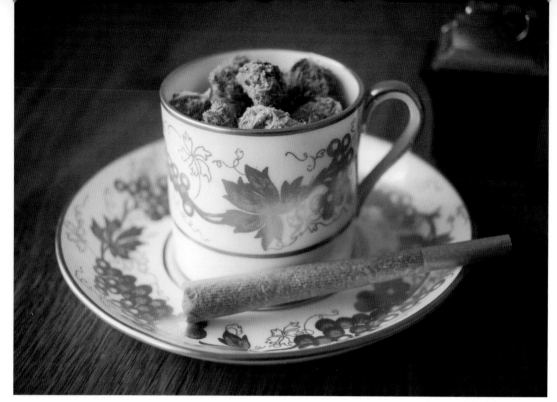

Because of the way artists tend to intertwine within each other's lives and work, a linear narrative of cannabis in art is difficult to capture succinctly, but here are a few of the major movements and players who helped define this notion of cannabis and creativity. Their belief and willingness to discuss and explore cannabis's positive uses in the open has helped advance societal understanding and acceptance of pot across generations. Artists are ambassadors who expand our collective comfort level and appreciation of cannabis.

Club des Hashischins

In the 1840s, a French doctor named Jacques Joseph Moreau experienced the **hashish** high on a trip to the Middle East and became obsessed with researching hash's effects. With the help of writer Pierre Jules Theophile Gautier, Moreau recruited a group of notable French authors and artists, including Honoré de Balzac, Victor Hugo, Gustave Flaubert, Eugène Delacroix, Gérard de Nerval, and Alexandre Dumas, to form The Hashish Club. Moreau was the first documented researcher to give cannabis to a group of creatives to explore their insights and experiences. In many ways, he was the forefather of this book. Moreau's approach was slightly more hands-on, but his gusto was admirable.

CANNABIS FOR CREATIVES

At their Parisian gatherings, some members of The Hashish Club would ingest a mixture of hash, sugar, and spices, while other members observed. Psychoactive experiences were the focus of the experimentation, and the writers were eager to find out how hash might inspire a creative impulse or expanded experience. Many of the members went on to write about their cannabis-fueled explorations or incorporate hash into famous works of fiction. In *The Count of Monte Cristo*, Dumas, inspired by his own experiences with hash, wrote, "Are you a man of imagination—a poet? Taste this, and the boundaries of possibility disappear; the fields of infinite space open to you, you advance free in heart, free in mind, into the boundless realms of unfettered reverie."

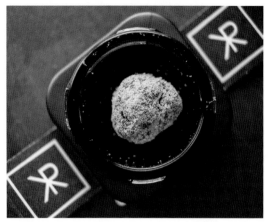

Moonrocks are a modern-day potent product that The Hashish Club would have loved, combining premium cannabis flower, hash oil, and **kief**.

The Birth of Jazz and the Death of Legal Cannabis in the US

Roughly 100 years later, one of America's best-known cannabis communities was born. Whether they called it "reefer," "tea," or "gage," the pioneers of jazz in New Orleans relied heavily on cannabis to fuel their music making. With a focus on improvisation, jazz musicians were drawn to cannabis for the way it seemed to expand time and add fluidity to their instrumentation. During the days of alcohol prohibition, smoking cannabis also offered an opportunity for many Black musicians to find some degree of mental relief from the anxieties and racial injustices they experienced living in the United States.

Louis Armstrong is perhaps the most well-known and outspoken pot-loving jazz musician, but other notable greats like Cab Calloway, Billie Holiday, Duke Ellington, Mezz Mezzrow, and Count Basie were all known to smoke cannabis before performances and recording sessions. Cannabis became a defining characteristic of the jazz movement, offering kinship, joy, relief, and the ability for artists to lose themselves in the music they loved.

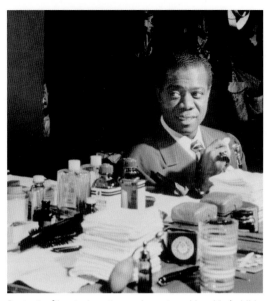

Portrait of Louis Armstrong, Aquarium, New York, NY, ca. July 1946, taken by William P. Gottlieb

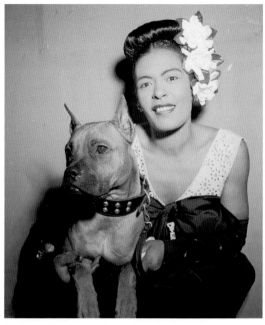

Portrait of Billie Holiday and Mister, Downbeat, New York, NY, ca. Feb. 1947, taken by William P. Gottlieb

Sadly, it's impossible to discuss the common and beneficial use of cannabis among Black jazz musicians without also addressing the way their pot use was weaponized through racist stereotypes depicting the dangers of pot. White politicians and government officials demonized jazz and pot use in equal measure, insisting that both would lead to the empowerment of Black members of the population and the corruption of white women and children. As alcohol prohibition ended, the US government, influenced largely by Harry J. Anslinger, commissioner for the Federal Bureau of Narcotics, needed somewhere else to direct their puritanical energy. They launched a full-scale propagandist war against cannabis.

Anslinger was a racist and a xenophobe with disastrous and far-reaching power and influence. Spend any time researching the man, and you'll see that he genuinely believed and spoke at length about white racial purity and superiority, regularly saying things like "…the primary reason to outlaw marijuana is its effect on the degenerate races.…"

Favoring the term *marijuana* for its Spanish-language origin, exotic sound, and the fear it would inspire in fellow xenophobes, Anslinger worked to convince white Americans that cannabis was a threat to their safety and to the delicate fabric of society. As a result of

CANNABIS FOR CREATIVES

his racist crusade, the Marihuana Tax Act of 1937 was passed and began a long, racially fueled tradition of prosecution and incarceration for the use, possession, and distribution of cannabis.

What began as a means for artists to seek mental relief and find new avenues of joy and creativity in their music indirectly resulted in the federal prohibition of cannabis that continues to this day.

Silver Screen and Green Buds

Jazz and the music scene of the 1920s, '30s, and '40s directly overlapped with a green wave among the actors of Hollywood's silver screen. In the decades that followed, many popular performers and cultural icons enjoyed cannabis both in their trailers and in their private lives.

In his notorious 1943 letter to the US troops stationed in Suriname, Groucho Marx wrote, "Last spring I was smart enough to plant a Victory garden. So far, I have raised a family of moles, enough snails to keep a pre-French restaurant running for a century and a curious

looking plant that I have been eating all summer under the impression that it was a vegetable. However, for the past few weeks, I've had difficulty in remaining awake and this morning I discovered that I had been munching on marijuana the whole month of July." In a television interview, Chico Marx explained that Groucho got his name for the "Grouch" bag he used to wear around his neck filled with miscellaneous items, including some cannabis.

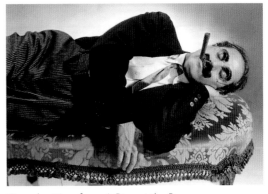

Groucho Marx from *A Day at the Races* (Photo by Ted Allan, for MGM, 1937)

While actor Robert Mitchum was outed as a cannabis smoker after his 1948 possession arrest and conviction, other Hollywood icons managed to keep their cannabis proclivities more private. Montgomery Clift, James Dean, Elizabeth Taylor, Tony Curtis, Steve McQueen, and Marilyn Monroe were among the many Hollywood stars rumored to enjoy cannabis, although the laws of the time prevented many of them from doing so openly.

While filming the 1969 movie *Easy Rider*, Dennis Hopper, Jack Nicholson, and Peter Fonda were reportedly smoking real cannabis onscreen. In a 2018 interview, Peter Fonda described how pivotal cannabis was in the scriptwriting process, saying, "When I was writing the story for *Easy Rider* and getting it all together and making my notes, I was stoned out of my gourd. I had a couple of **doobies**, and I think a couple of bottles of Heineken. So I was feeling no pain, and the story just flowed out of me."

Counterculture Movements of the 1960s and 1970s

Easy Rider, and its anti-propagandist stance on drugs was made possible in many ways by the cultural movements of the decade that preceded it. The 1960s represented the beginning of a massive cultural shift that reverberates even now. Feminism, the civil rights movement, the sexual revolution, gay liberation, opposition to the Vietnam War, hippies, and beatniks challenged the authority of the government, the white-male-run establishment, and the blanket vilification of drugs and alternative lifestyles. While these movements focused on a variety of individual goals, cannabis use was a common thread for many, present at protests and meetings and helping to unify and embolden those who challenged the status quo.

In 1966, Allen Ginsberg, poet and one of the defining voices of his generation, wrote an essay for *The Atlantic* called "The Great Marijuana Hoax: First Manifesto to End the Bringdown." In the essay, Ginsberg called out Anslinger for his moralistic, racist, and deeply inaccurate portrayals of cannabis and cannabis users. To educate the masses and challenge anti-cannabis sentiment, he spoke directly to those who had never personally experienced pot, expressing cannabis's ability to expand the mind and the senses to provide insights. For his efforts, Ginsberg was awarded a thick government file and a heightened level of federal scrutiny for the duration of his life.

Allen Ginsberg wasn't the only member of the community known as the Beat Generation to find value in psychoactive substances. Frustrated by bureaucratic lies, writers like William S. Burroughs, Jack Kerouac, and Neal Cassady held pro-pot rallies, wrote expansive works fueled by and focusing on mind-altering substances, and fought to change the cultural narrative surrounding cannabis. In discussing his process, Burroughs famously said, "Unquestionably, this drug is very useful to the artist, activating trains of association that would otherwise be inaccessible, and I owe many of the scenes in *Naked Lunch* directly to the use of cannabis."

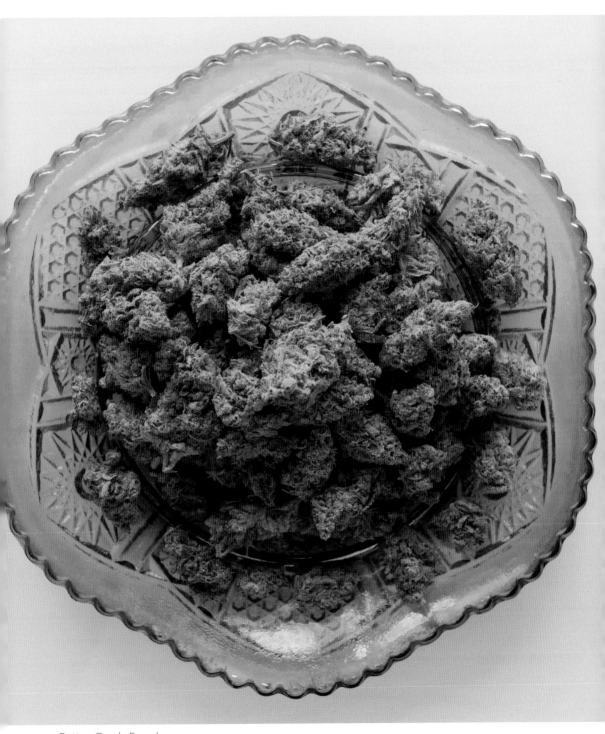

Cotton Candy Romulan

Visionaries with high hopes for the future of society, many of them artists themselves, found comfort and clarity in cannabis, even while Richard Nixon launched the War on Drugs. Determined to vilify and prosecute the use of mind-altering substances, Nixon consolidated and expanded federal agencies focusing on drug control and ignored a federal commission recommending decriminalization of cannabis possession. Years later, John Ehrlichman, a Nixon aide, admitted that the war on drugs was created to penalize the anti-war hippie and Black communities, but a precedent was set in both government and conservative public opinion. An increasing divide grew between straightlaced, conservative communities and the cannabis-loving baby boomers. Artists like Cheech & Chong, who are hilarious to those who love cannabis, also seemed to reinforce the ferocity of anti-cannabis sentiments among its opponents.

Hip-Hop and the Return to the Mainstream

In the 1980s, Ronald Reagan expanded many of Nixon's drug laws while Nancy Reagan introduced the "Just Say No" campaign. What was presented by America's first couple as an attempt to keep citizens safe from the dangers of drug use further fueled racial disparity, increased penalties for cannabis possession, and instituted harsh mandatory minimum sentences.

Artists like Peter Tosh, Bob Marley, Rick James, George Clinton, and other icons in reggae, funk, and R & B, had been singing openly about cannabis for years, paving the way for early DJs and hip-hop artists to respond directly to America's anti-drug campaigns and legislation. Rappers used their growing platform and notoriety to lead conversations about cannabis and normalize getting high. Passing references evolved into a major topic of musical conversation. Tupac Shakur, Biggie Smalls, Dr. Dre, Cypress Hill, Snoop Dogg, OutKast, and Wu-Tang Clan were just a few of the visionaries responsible for a cultural shift in transparency and appreciation of cannabis. They presented smoking pot as a totally normal, harmless, and enjoyable way of life, providing relief from stress and building a sense of community. In many ways, the rise of hip-hop combined the musical value and social escape felt by pot-smoking jazz musicians with the audacity and cultural commentary that defined the 1960s counterculture. Hip-hop artists became the spokespersons for a new generation of cannabis enthusiasts, speaking openly not just about pot's positive qualities but about the hypocrisy and disproportionate drug prosecution in Black communities.

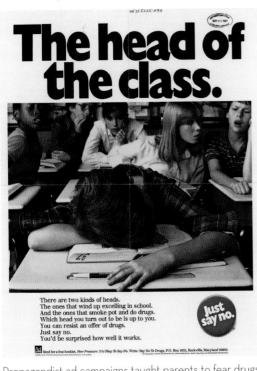

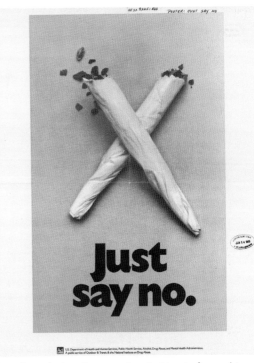

Propagandist ad campaigns taught parents to fear drugs and reinforced a long-lasting cultural mistrust of cannabis.

As hip-hop grew in popularity, the modern culture of cannabis also grew. Lyrics drew a distinct line between pot and other drugs as legislation in California endeavored to do the same. Icons of the genre used their popularity and voice to sway public opinion and bring cannabis use to the mainstream. It took time, but it worked. We simply wouldn't be where we are now if not for them.

A Shared Heritage in Creativity

Building on a foundation of insights and explorations of artistic generations that came before us, contemporary artists continue to look to cannabis as a source of expanded thought and unbridled access to inner creative streams. While movements like the birth of jazz stand out as representative and defining moments in the American story of cannabis, artists around the world and throughout other creative eras have successfully utilized pot for their artistic processes. Diego Rivera, the Beatles, Jimi Hendrix, Salvador Dalí, Ernest Hemingway, George Carlin, Dave Chappelle, Seth Rogen, Carl Sagan, Bob Dylan, Willie Nelson, and

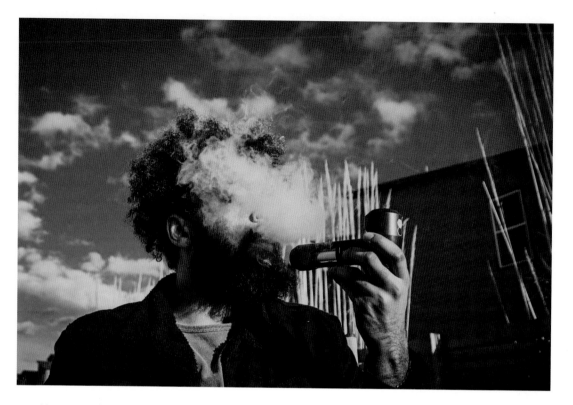

Hunter S. Thompson are just a few of the many influential artists who have found comfort and inspiration in pot.

For these artists, and countless others, cannabis represents a means of counteracting external and internal pressures. Judgement, doubt, perfectionism, and fear are navigated and surpassed. Ideas emerge, clarify, and take concrete form. Smoking pot can be a means of escape from restrictions of the mind, a synthesizer of community, and a source of joy. For outspoken critics like Anslinger, Richard Nixon, and Ronald Reagan, stoned thinking is a detriment, but at its core, stoned thinking is a method of problem solving and philosophy building uninhibited by self-made and culturally initiated roadblocks or bounds of traditional thought.

CHAPTER 2

STUDYING CREATIVITY

Medicine and science have come a long way in recent years. We can 3D print body parts for rejection-proof transplants, perform complex surgeries with help from robots, and predict medical predispositions with blood tests. Yet, even with all that we've learned, the brain remains one of the most elusive parts of the human body.

We used to believe that the left and right hemispheres of the brain were individually responsible for different tasks and functions. You'd hear, "She's so left brained" to describe someone who is analytical or "He's definitely right brained" to describe someone who is more creative, but in recent years we've shifted away from that dual-hemisphere representation.

Rather than examining hemispheres or even distinct brain structures, like the amygdala or the hippocampus, to explain systemic activities and behaviors, we now look at brain networks. Individual structures have their roles, but science places greater emphasis on how structures work together to achieve various functions. Think of it this way: a car doesn't accelerate solely because of its spark plugs. Sure, spark plugs are important and play their role, but the car accelerates because of how the spark plugs work in concert with hundreds of other engine components.

Understanding the brain networks and how they interact with each other and the rest of the body is vital for understanding important functions of life, from things like emotions and the fight-or-flight response, to hormone regulation and sensations of hunger.

Which Brain Networks Are Involved in Creativity?

To understand creativity, many studies focus on three key brain networks: the *default mode network*, the *executive attention network*, and the *salience network*. These networks aren't limited to creativity or activities related to creativity. They're deeply ingrained in many parts of our existence, but when examining creativity specifically, they are the key players.

The Default Mode Network

Frequently referred to as the imagination network, the default mode network relates to activities that involve inward thinking. When you create a new personal goal, reflect introspectively about a project you're working on, or try to imagine a situation from another person's perspective, you're using the default mode network.

When it comes to creative pursuits, the default mode network is vital. Brainstorming ideas, considering hypothetical problems or solutions, and looser, uninhibited thoughts originate here. Without these capabilities, we'd be stuck writing the same songs over and over or repainting Vincent van Gogh's *The Starry Night* simply because we couldn't come up with our own ideas and inspiration.

How many times have you started a project related to big-C Creativity or little-c creativity with a brainstorm session? You can thank your default mode network for the ideas you generated, both amazing and terrible.

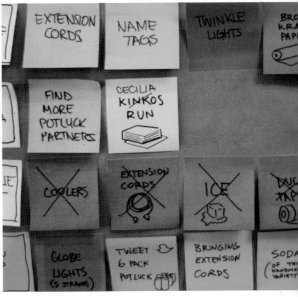

Brainstorming in art and in life utilizes our default mode network.

The Executive Attention Network

Also known as the executive functioning network, this brain network relates to functions and activities handled with a greater depth of focus. When you follow an idea down a rabbit hole, develop a strategy to solve a problem, or refer to your working memory to see how situations compare to problems and solutions of the past, you're using the executive attention network.

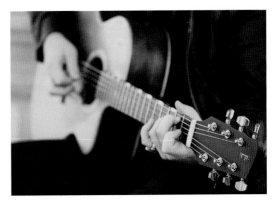

Learning a tricky guitar part (or writing one) requires the kind of focus that only the executive attention network can provide.

Creative pursuits rely heavily on the executive attention network. It takes charge when we explore ideas in more depth and limits how much attention we devote to pursuing the most obvious ideas. It's how we identify and explore concepts with a greater potential for success.

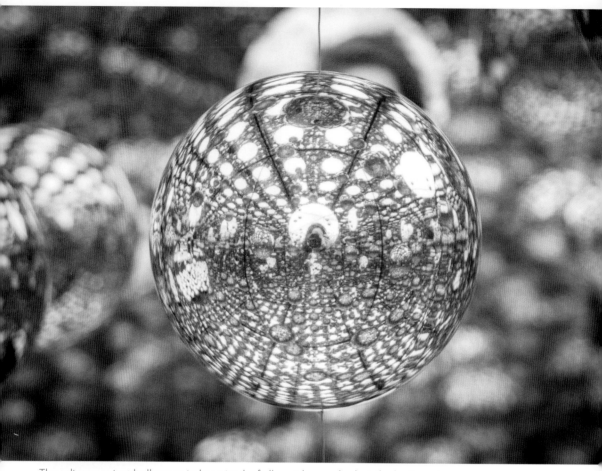

The salience network allows us to keep track of all our ideas and select the best one to pursue.

When you maintain hyper focus on a project, effectively tuning out lesser ideas and distractions, or become deeply engaged in a complex task, you have your executive attention network to thank. Most creatives require and value this aspect of their brains when working in depth on a project, whether it's writing lyrics to a song, composing a detailed photograph, or cooking a complicated dish.

The executive attention network also relates to another vital aspect of the creative process: self-awareness and self-consciousness. Most people (hopefully) have some sense of self-awareness, and in the world of creativity, we are often our own harshest critics. The executive attention network is responsible when we feel satisfied or dissatisfied with a project or performance.

The Salience Network

Acting as a switching station, the salience network determines when to transfer activity between the default mode network and the executive attention network. Without a functioning salience network, we wouldn't know when to keep brainstorming and when to pick an idea and move forward into more concentrated concept development.

Our salience network helps our creative ideas progress, so we can modulate our focus as we come up with ideas and develop them further.

When a painter looks at a scene and decides what part of it to paint, the salience network is responsible for making that selection. It helps label ideas and stimuli as either interesting or not worth exploring. The salience network is vital in balancing our present experiences and our memories of the past to adapt and modify our behavior and thoughts.

How Brain Networks Work Together

So, what are the practical uses of these networks for diverse types of creative thought and work? Here are two examples of how artists use each of these networks as they develop their ideas and create art:

The Photographer

A photographer looks at a natural landscape. We'll call her Jordana because that's a fine name for a photographer to have. Jordana sees a broad vista with mountains in the distance, bands of forest, and wildflowers at her feet. Looking at the scene in front of her, she uses her default mode network to run through ideas of potential photos she could take. She envisions panoramas, a couple close-ups of flowers, and maybe a long exposure to capture the movement of the clouds above. She brainstorms all these possible shots.

Using her salience network, she decides that she wants to photograph the wider image first because it feels like it might be the strongest choice, just in case she runs out of time or the light changes.

Shifting to her executive attention network, she sets up her tripod, grabs her wide-angle lens, and adjusts her aperture to best capture the scene.

Jordana shoots a few images, making slight variations based on the memories of past successes and failures with similar landscapes and lighting scenarios (executive attention network). She checks her shots with an eye for self-evaluation (executive attention network) and decides to adjust her settings and composition based on how she wants her viewers to understand and engage with the scene (salience network switching to default mode network). She focuses on the new composition and concentrates on getting her ideal shot (executive attention network).

Later, at the computer, Jordana looks at all the images she took and picks a favorite to develop (salience network). She considers all the potential ways of developing the image (default mode network) before choosing the look that best benefits the image (salience network). Finally, she spends some time perfecting the shot (executive functioning network).

The Comedic Improv Actors

Two improv actors (we'll call them Ben and Tom) are onstage, ready to begin a new improvisational scene. Ben internally brainstorms great scene concepts using his default mode network. He settles on "things you might overhear in a doctor's office," which his salience network identifies as a potentially hilarious direction to take the scene. He asks the audience to help brainstorm appropriate phrases (now Ben engages the audience's default mode networks too).

As audience members shout out phrases, his salience network remains active, listening to all the suggestions and determining the best options for use in the scene. He chooses his favorite and is ready to begin.

Shifting to his default mode network to explore his favorite suggestion further, he turns to his scene partner and pantomimes pulling down his pants. Now, imagining his rear to be exposed (default mode network), Ben utters his favorite audience suggestion: "Does this look normal to you?"

What follows is a long and hilarious exploration utilizing multiple brain networks. Ben and Tom constantly switch between their default mode and executive attention networks to take jokes farther, gauge audience response, and adapt the scene. All the while, they're relying on their salience networks to serve as the switching station, indicating when it's time for more brainstorming or self-reflection, or when it's time to take a joke farther.

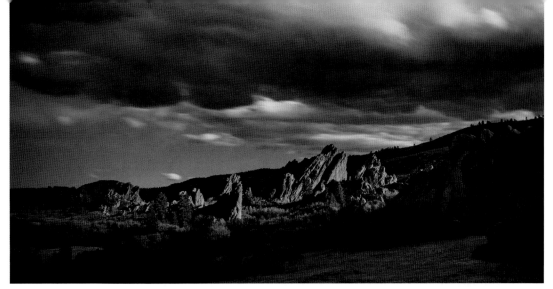

Making a successful photograph involves seamlessly switching back and forth between brain networks.

Improvisation, or any live work in front of an audience, keeps all three of these brain networks active because artists must constantly adapt based on audience response and self-evaluation of success.

Creative pursuits of any variety are an ongoing juggling act. As artists, we constantly switch from one dominant brain network to another and back again. In most cases, we do this seamlessly and without paying any particular attention to what's happening along the way. Some creative processes require more use of one network over another. Different tasks demand different parts of our brains, and for different durations.

Some scientific studies have suggested that creative people are better equipped to readily switch between one network and another or to use multiple networks simultaneously. For many, it's as natural a process as getting dressed or brushing our teeth, and yet we rarely stop to consider what exactly is happening in our brains.

How Does Science Measure Creativity?

Neuroscience and psychology suggest a distinct relationship between our ability to successfully function in life and the use of these brain networks. While the average person might not consider the daily impact of brain networks on their life, scientists want to understand each network and how they are used in creative activities. They attempt to do so through a variety of standardized tests and exploratory studies. But before you can study something, you must decide how to measure it.

Try to think of a quantifiable way of measuring creativity. The method must require few supplies and be easy to replicate in schools or doctors' offices. Ideally it should be a task that a person of any age or educational background can perform. Any luck?

It's quite difficult to conceive of the perfect test, whether you're concerned with practical little-c creativity, artsy big-C Creativity, or both. Psychologists currently use a series of standardized tests with the intention of assessing creativity levels. These tests aren't perfect, and generally they're geared more toward measuring little-c creativity, but they are relatively easy to replicate in multiple environments and with subjects of any age.

Divergent Thinking vs. Convergent Thinking

Scientifically, creativity is most commonly measured in terms of divergent thinking and convergent thinking. Through standardized tests using word problems and scenarios, divergent and convergent thinking is fairly quantifiable. Tests can be scored uniformly, and test takers can be ranked against their peers. But what exactly are divergent and convergent thinking, and how do they relate to concepts of creativity?

Divergent Thinking in Creativity

Divergent thinking specifically relates to idea generation stemming from exploring multiple possible ideas and outcomes. Brainstorming, for example, is all about divergent thinking. Employers love divergent thinkers for their ability to problem solve in real-life scenarios.

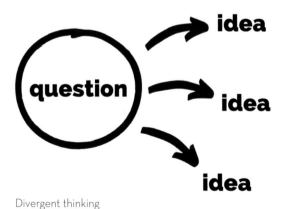

Divergent thinking

The complication in quantifying creativity using divergent thinking assessments is that there are no "right" answers. Divergent thinking tends to be subjective. If I ask two different people to brainstorm uses for a brick, they will each have a distinct set of responses based on their life experiences.

The Alternate Uses Task (AUT) is a test that does just that. Test subjects are asked to list as many uses for an object as possible in two minutes. Let's stick with the brick as an example. Officially, a brick is used as a building material, but it can also be used as a doorstop, a water conservation tool in a toilet tank, a free weight, a landscaping border, and a weapon. If you wanted to get really crazy, you could use a brick like a pumice stone to remove dead skin, as a meat tenderizer, or you could use it as an anchor for a very small boat. In the AUT, each of these suggested uses would be measured and scored for fluency (quantity), originality, flexibility (how wide ranging in scope the ideas are), and elaboration (how developed each idea is).

If you're wondering how there can possibly be a consistent scoring rubric for something as subjective as determining originality, you're not alone. This test also connotes speed and success. When was the last time you demonstrated the depth of your creativity in under two minutes? Tests like the AUT are great for identifying both extremes on a spectrum—subjects who are wildly creative or who have very limited creative capabilities—but they're not quite as nuanced as one might hope for understanding Creativity.

Think about art as it relates to divergent thinking. A chef could utilize divergent thinking to find other ways of using a common ingredient, or a photographer could incorporate it by finding a new use for a certain lens. Beyond brainstorming, divergent thinking has many similarities with the processes utilized by the default mode network. So, especially as it relates to originality, divergent thinking is an especially useful skill for a creative person to possess, regardless of how difficult it may be to accurately measure.

Convergent Thinking in Creativity

Convergent thinking relates to finding the best possible solution for a set of criteria. The multiple-choice tests we grew up taking in school require successful convergent thinking (and sometimes luck). This type of thought process has endless real-life applications in the world of little-c creativity. When you're overdue for a grocery run and still manage to make an appetizing dinner out of a random assortment of ingredients and condiments left in the fridge, you're practicing convergent thinking.

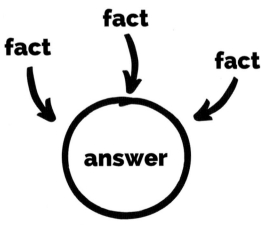

Convergent thinking

When it comes to testing for convergent thinking, the results are much more objective. Compared to the fluidity of divergent thinking concepts, convergent thinking is easier to quantify.

The Remote Associates Test (RAT) is a common assessment tool for measuring convergent thinking. Subjects receive a list of words that seem unrelated until they are linked with an additional commonly associated word.

Here's a simple example: cloth, puff, and grater. What word could be commonly associated with each of those? The answer is "cheese." Cheese cloth, cheese puff, and cheese grater.

This next example is a bit harder: right, carbon, cat. The answer is "copy." Copyright, carbon copy, copycat.

The RAT is easier to grade than the AUT because there's usually only one correct answer for each collection of words. It's logic-based and finite. If you're fluent in the language used on the test, you should score well.

Practical applications of convergent thinking in art aren't quite as obvious. Chefs can use convergent thinking to create recipes with available ingredients, but convergent thinking for actors, musicians, and visual artists is harder to identify, especially when viewed within the criteria of the RAT.

Convergent thinking is somewhat related to the executive functioning network and the salience network, but it's far more applicable to little c-creativity and functioning in the workplace than it is to generating artistic output.

Measuring Creativity After Cannabis Use

Many of the same types of tests used to assess creativity in terms of divergent and convergent thinking have been given to cannabis users over the years to determine whether cannabis is enhancing or impairing creativity.

A 2014 study called "Cannabis and creativity: highly potent cannabis impairs divergent thinking in regular cannabis users," is one example of an endeavor to empirically determine whether a connection between cannabis and creativity exists. The double-blind study was performed in the Netherlands where there are fewer governmental limitations for studying cannabis. Fifty-four participants randomly received one of three doses: a placebo in the form of a cannabis look-alike that contained no THC or other psychoactive ingredients, a 5.5-mg dose of THC, or a 22-mg dose of THC. The doses were administered via a Volcano **vaporizer**.

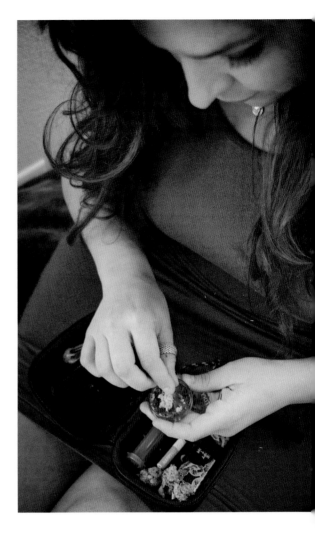

The Random Associates Test (RAT) and the Alternate Uses Task (AUT) were administered as the official means of measuring creativity. Participants who received a 5.5-mg dosage performed slightly better on the AUT than the placebo group in terms of fluency and flexibility of ideas, and significantly better than the placebo group in terms of originality of ideas. But in each of those three categories (fluency, flexibility, and originality), the 22-mg dosage group performed comparatively poorly. The results of the convergent thinking-based RAT didn't demonstrate any significant differences, so it didn't weigh into the study's findings.

What does that mean? At face value, this study demonstrates that some aspects of divergent thinking improve with lower doses of THC. It also suggests that higher doses of THC can interfere with those same aspects of divergent thinking. So, smoke a little bit and you can amplify creativity. Smoke a bunch and you might be doing more harm than good to your creative flow.

Like many scientific cannabis studies, this one has some flaws. The most glaring concern is that only one strain of cannabis, Bedrocan, was administered. This study may provide

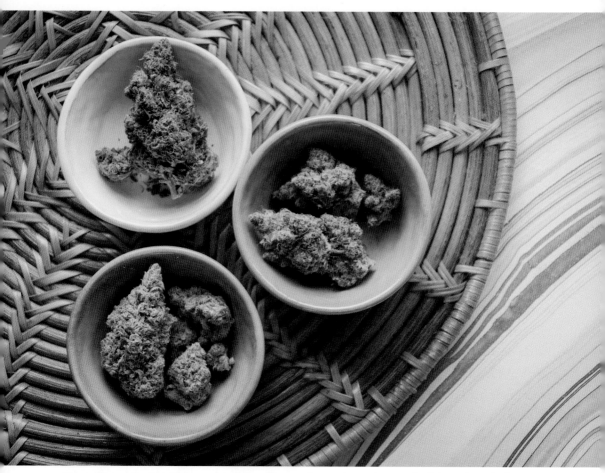

There are practically infinite combinations of types of cannabis and ways of imbibing. A study that examines only one variety or method can't possibly define all user experiences.

insights about Bedrocan use, but does it speak to the hundreds of other cannabis strains or to cannabis as a psychoactive substance in general? Not really. Add to that the questionable logic of using AUT and RAT scores to reflect real-world creativity, and this study, like so many others along the same vein, isn't quite as representative as scientists might hope.

These limitations aren't being mentioned to shame researchers or call into question the efficacy of studying pot in a lab, it's merely to highlight just how complex these issues are. If we're going to base click-bait headlines, public opinion, and legislation on these sorts of findings, the approach needs to be more balanced and wide-ranging.

Qualitative vs. Quantitative Reflections on Cannabis and Creativity

If lab testing and quantitative assessments are so flawed, why do we keep placing so much value in them? Well, scientists, doctors, and governments tend to prefer hard numbers. I could tell you that most of my friends smoke weed, or I could tell you that I've polled my friends and 72% of them smoke weed. Which of those statements feels more tangible? More concrete?

When it comes to defining trends, approving medications, and creating legislation, we gravitate toward verifiable statistics over personal accounts and anecdotes. Numbers feel more real. But having reflected on some of the more imprecise aspects of these studies, the numbers, with all their limitations, don't seem sufficient.

I spoke with Josh Kaplan, Ph.D., Professor of Behavioral Neuroscience at Western Washington University, and frequent contributor to *High Times* and *Leafly*. He reiterated some of the complications he's seen in previous lab studies related to cannabis and its effects:

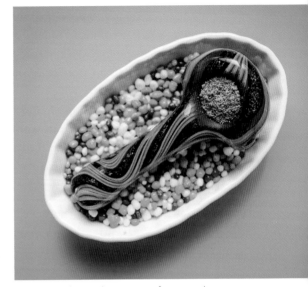

Most cannabis enthusiasts prefer pipes, bongs, joints, edibles, or a wide variety of other methods. IV injected THC isn't realistic outside of a lab.

When we're looking at studies conducted in a laboratory setting, all of the information that's known about cannabis is derived from just a select few sources. Often, we're talking about either isolated THC or almost 99% THC, which is not what you would get in a traditional flower, which might have 10–30% THC. Even in the rare cases where flower is tested, it's typically not a strain anyone is using recreationally or medicinally. It's a very limited scientific approach. It doesn't necessarily model human use patterns and that's a major problem. In a lot of studies from the '70s and '80s, and even some from the '90s, they're studying IV-injected THC to control for dosing. I've never seen anyone IV inject THC. That has very different pharmacokinetic properties than smoking it, or vaping, or eating a brownie. You read about these studies of THC-induced psychosis and other things. Is that gonna happen in a real world setting at the rate and extent that you're reading about in these studies? My hypothesis would be no. From observation, no.

What about the efficacy of studying creativity by measuring divergent and convergent thinking? I expressed my frustration with boiling such an amorphous concept as creativity into these very regimented, specific tasks and trying to make broad characterizations about cannabis and creativity. Dr. Kaplan sympathized with my misgivings:

> *I think researchers recognize that there are challenges, because you're right: creativity, when it comes to music, it involves more than just divergent thinking if it involves timing. With music, timing is such a key thing. We know that cannabis, and THC in particular, makes people overestimate the amount of time that has passed, which means that their perception of time is slowing. Those types of divergent and convergent measures aren't taking into account this kind of sensory perception. In the case of a chef or a musician or someone who requires all of that sensory input, now that's enhanced. That could contribute to creativity in the arts and it wouldn't be captured by that type of measure.*

The combination of governmental bottlenecks and incomplete or ineffective standardized assessments of creativity make quantitative studies and data sets hard to justify in the pursuit of understanding the complex relationship between cannabis and creativity. This is why qualitative data is so deeply relevant as a supplemental source of information.

In his book *The Natural Mind*, Dr. Andrew Weil presents a similar set of concerns and caveats about lab research, concluding, "Laboratory information is interesting and has its place, but the only ultimately valid source of information is direct experience." Dr. Mitch Earleywine, author of *Understanding Marijuana*, agrees, saying he's read, "page after page of laboratory studies with methodological issues. There seems to be no way to empirically study the effects of pot—so we'll rely on the anecdotal."

Interview Methodologies

When I decided to approach creatives about their cannabis use, I had my work cut out for me. As much as pot enthusiasts love the stuff, not everyone wants to go on record about it (a handful agreed to an interview under the condition of anonymity). Interested in expanding my scope as far as age range, home state or country, cultural background, type of art, and

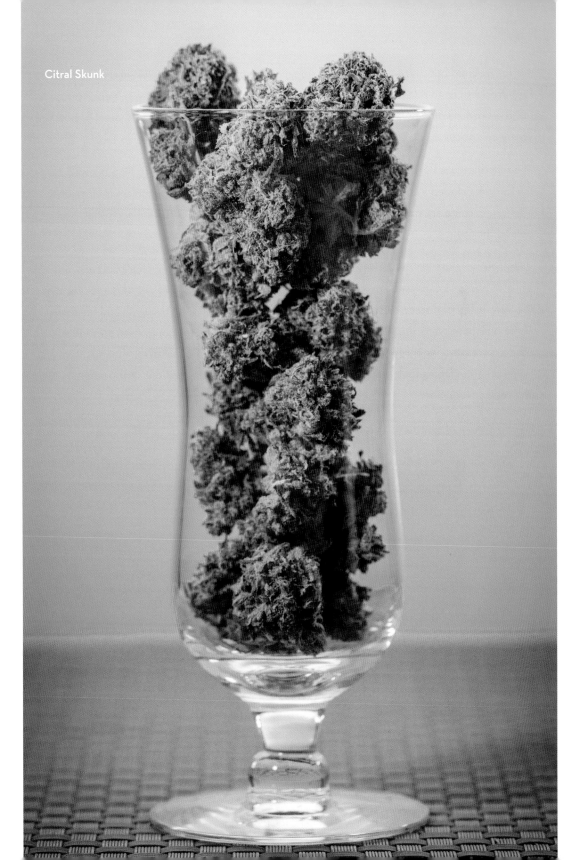

Citral Skunk

more, I reached out to friends and professional contacts asking not only for interviews but for introductions to relevant creatives who might have some insights on the subject. I put out a sponsored post on Instagram as well as a series of publicly visible and shareable posts on my own social media pages.

The response was significant. I originally intended to speak to 10 to 12 artists. I interviewed 32. My sample included a range of artists who work with a variety of media. Some are professional artists, and some are hobbyists. Some work on the front end of art creation and others work behind the scenes.

All but two of the interviews were held over video chat. One was a phone call, and one was a live, in-person interview. I approached all my interviews with the same set of questions, but the informality of the conversational setting often led to meandering thoughts and tangents. Some questions were answered organically by the subjects before I could even ask, while others were never concretely pinned down. That's the beauty of qualitative research. It's a living, breathing thing that changes shape as needed to suit the conditions of the subject and the conversation.

Here is the list of questions I brought to each interview:

- Can you give me a little background on your artistic journey?
- When did cannabis come into your life?
- Do you think cannabis makes you more creative?
- When/how did you discover that cannabis influenced your creative process?
- Walk me through your process; is it always the same?
- Do you imbibe when you intend to create, or is creation an occasional byproduct?
- Why do you think cannabis makes you more creative?
- What does the cannabis-inspired creative energy feel like?
- What other pathways or creative rituals do you employ?
- Does a specific strain or method matter for your creative response?
- Does your creative process change if you don't imbibe?
- Is your creative process solo or communal?
- Does your creativity depend on cannabis?

In reading these questions, you may notice that my approach presupposes a relationship between cannabis and creativity. As a cannabis user myself, I inevitably view the conversation with my own set of unavoidable biases. Dr. Andrew Weil accurately addressed this inherent issue when he wrote, "Everyone who speaks or writes about drugs (and certainly all who 'investigate' them) together with everyone who hears or reads what is said and written has an emotional involvement with the information. The exact nature of this involvement differs from person to person in both degree and quality, but it is always there." In essence, bias is unavoidable. I have my own bias toward cannabis, which is different from yours, which is different from a DEA agent's bias. We recognize that the bias exists and move on.

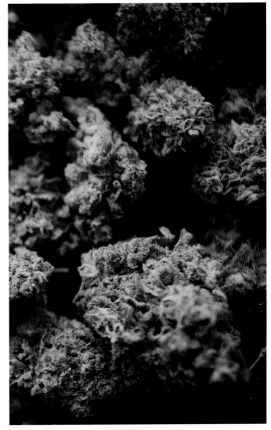

Flo

By contacting creative cannabis users, I specifically targeted a group of people who have already formed opinions about cannabis and art-making. This book was conceived from my presupposition that there is a relationship. Through each of the interviews, I was able to adapt and expand my understanding of that relationship.

All interviews were recorded and transcribed for more precise review and analysis. In later chapters, you'll read a combination of short quotes and longer discussions from the interviews. They have all been edited for clarity and length, but the essence of each reported experience is authentic and unchanged.

One of the surprising outcomes of my research is seeing just how varied our experiences with cannabis are. As you read the interviews, you'll find that some artists have much more defined effects related to their default mode network, while others chase that executive functioning network rabbit hole to the very end.

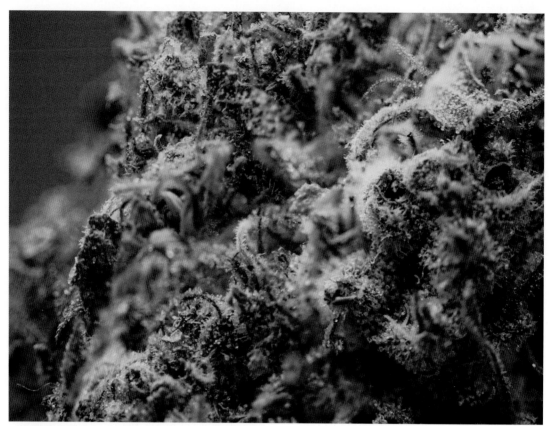

Chocolope

In the greater pursuit of understanding how cannabis and creativity relate, there's certainly a place in the discussion for laboratory studies, but many cannabis enthusiasts are already doing the trial-and-error research for themselves. Their insights and experiences can help unlock the potential of cannabis use not only for creativity, but for a happier, more productive life.

CHAPTER 3

CANNABIS AND THE BRAIN

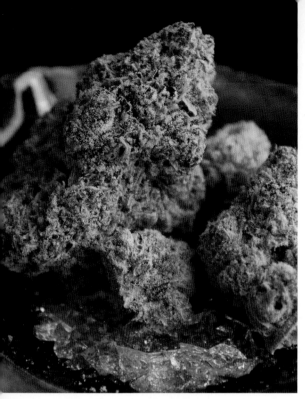

Deep Chunk

What exactly happens in the brain when we smoke a joint or eat a pot gummy? Well, it's complex. Cannabis, as we'll discuss in detail later, contains over 100 chemical compounds called **cannabinoids**. These chemicals exist in different quantities and different combinations from one strain of cannabis to another. That's one of the reasons why it's so difficult to make blanket statements about what cannabis does and doesn't do to our bodies and minds. Each strain is different.

We're mostly interested in tetrahydro-cannabinol (THC, also known as delta-9-THC) because it's the primary psychoactive ingredient found in cannabis. THC and other cannabinoids interact with a natural system in the body called the **endocannabinoid system**. When we smoke, the endocannabinoid system is what allows our body to respond to pot. It's responsible for the feelings of euphoria, pain relief, hunger, and other general concepts of being "high."

The Endocannabinoid System

The human body and all its components function like a well-oiled machine. Much like the networks of the brain work together to fuel creative thought, the systems of the body perform a constant ebb and flow of signals and responses.

Among the structures allowing our survival is the endocannabinoid system. In my younger, less researched years, I naively believed that this meant there was a part of my body that nature had developed purely for the ability to recognize and be affected by pot. It's a common misconception, and it makes sense. If I had a receptor that scientists had dubbed "the bark mulch acceptance system," I might believe that some part of my body was designed to metabolize bark mulch.

In actuality, the endocannabinoid system got its name because researchers first discovered it while studying the response to cannabis in test subjects. Rather than name the receptors for their original biological functions (which they hadn't yet determined), they named the receptors for the psychoactive substance that makes use of them. It's a backward way of addressing things, but here we are.

The endocannabinoid system includes three main components: endocannabinoid receptors, endocannabinoids, and metabolic enzymes.

Endocannabinoid receptors exist throughout the brain and body. There are two specific types of receptors, CB1 and CB2, named for the order in which they were discovered. CB1 receptors are found in the brain and a few other locations throughout the body and are receptive to the psychoactive and mood-enhancing properties of cannabis. They also play a part in pain relief. CB2 receptors, located throughout the body, don't respond to

psychoactive elements of cannabis, but they do relate to inflammatory response, pain processing, and the immune system, some of the other common benefits cited by cannabis enthusiasts.

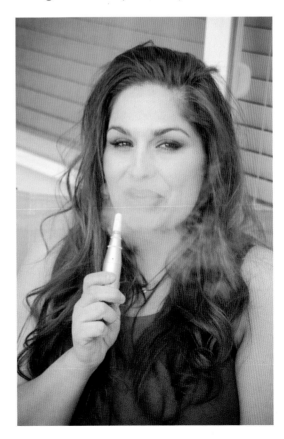

Endocannabinoids are chemicals produced *endogenously*, or naturally, by the body to interact with endocannabinoid receptors. The two endocannabinoids that we currently know about are Anandamide and 2-Arachidonoylglycerol (2-AG).

Anandamide, named for the Sanskrit word *ananda*, meaning "bliss," has a variety of uses in the human body. It's related to decreasing fear or anxiety, increasing appetite, and slowing activity. It's also believed to be related to memory, motor functions, and perception of pain. You might be wondering why, if your body naturally produces an endocannabinoid with these effects, you don't feel high all the time. Well, the body produces chemicals like anandamide as needed, and they don't stick around in our systems for nearly as long as external cannabinoids. They appear when required to maintain homeostasis, and they break down fairly quickly, having achieved their goals.

2-AG, our other endocannabinoid, interacts with both CB1 and CB2 receptors, and is associated with nausea suppression, pain relief, and inhibition of tumor growth, which relates to why cannabis is so popular among cancer patients.

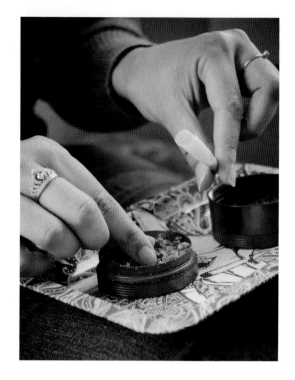

CB1 receptors are found throughout the portions of the brain involved in the executive attention network, the salience network, and the default mode network. As we toke, we're directly introducing an *exogenous* (or externally sourced) cannabinoid to areas that are deeply related to the creative process.

What Happens in the Brain When We Get High?

Brain cells communicate with each other by releasing chemicals called neurotransmitters. Those neurotransmitters jump from an upstream neuron across a gap, called a synaptic cleft, where they are received by downstream neurons. In most neurons, the flow of information is one directional, from upstream to downstream.

In the endocannabinoid system, the communication between neurons flows both directions. When upstream neurons are overly active, they trigger downstream neurons to release endocannabinoids. This helps quiet the overactive upstream neurons. Those endocannabinoids are sent back across the synaptic cleft to be received by the upstream neuron's endocannabinoid receptors.

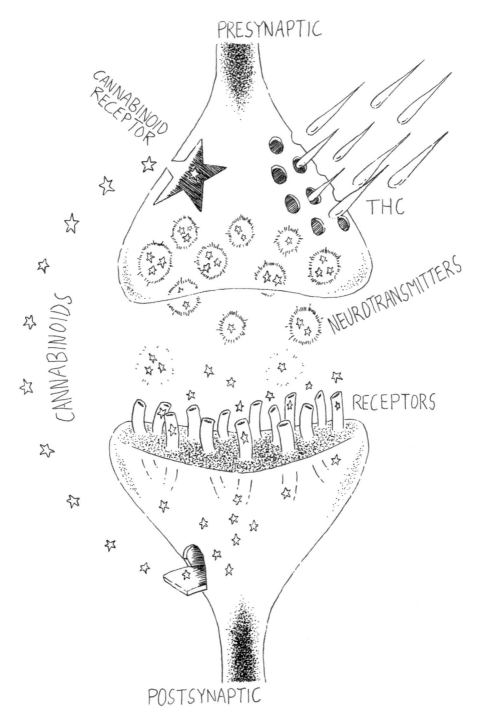

PRESYNAPTIC

CANNABINOID RECEPTOR

THC

CANNABINOIDS

NEUROTRANSMITTERS

RECEPTORS

POSTSYNAPTIC

The endocannabinoid system responds to both endogenous cannabinoids like anandamide and exogenous ones like THC. (Illustration by John McAmis)

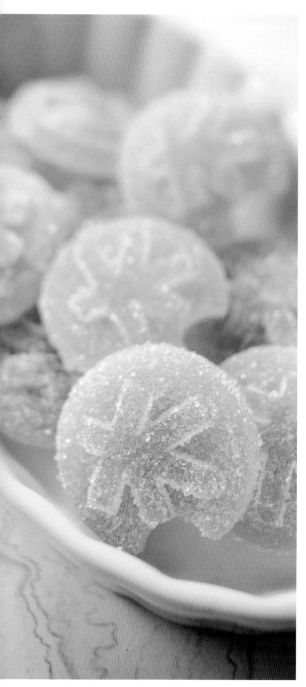

Here's where things get a bit more complicated: in some parts of the brain, neurons are *excitatory*, meaning that their activation results in greater levels of activity, and some are *inhibitory*, meaning that their activation dampens levels of activity. If you think of the system like a light switch, an excitatory neuron becoming activated would turn on the light. An inhibitory neuron becoming activated would turn off the light.

The external cannabinoids we introduce into our systems, whether via inhalation, ingestion, or other means, activate those upstream neurons via their cannabinoid receptors. Unlike our naturally occurring endocannabinoids, these exogenous chemicals interact indiscriminately and are relatively long lasting. Various parts of the brain deal with that cannabinoid interference differently. Excitatory neurons are prevented from initiating their traditional activities, while inhibitory neurons are prevented from causing their dampening activities. So, smoking pot can keep excitatory neurons from flipping the switch on, and it can prevent inhibitory neurons from flipping the switch off.

Sour Berry Bombs and other cannabis products introduce exogenous cannabinoids into our bodies.

For example, Dr. Josh Kaplan presented how introducing cannabinoids can relate to feelings of anxiety:

> One person might smoke some weed and they say, 'Hey, that helps me feel calm.' That could be in part because it's reducing the output of a brain region known as the amygdala, which is part of our threat detection system. It gets a little haywire when we're feeling anxious and stressed. But when people smoke too much and they get too high, then they feel more anxious because it's increasing the output of that area. It's also working to dampen the output of other areas, like the prefrontal cortex. So working memory and executive functioning are impaired when we are too stoned.

This sort of region-specific variability makes it very difficult to make overgeneralizations about the effects of THC and other cannabinoids on the brain, adding to the need for further uninhibited research with real-world use cases.

What Does It Feel Like?

When I smoke (my preferred method) cannabis flower, I can experience a wide range of effects depending on the strain, my environment, how much I smoke, and my preexisting mental state. Generally, smoking pot relaxes me, clarifies my thoughts, and makes me feel more lighthearted and silly. I like energetic strains and the feeling of inspiration and motivation they bring. They seem to drive my inner energy outward, manifesting in activity and productivity. Sometimes the hyperfocus I experience leads me to notice details and beauty where it might not normally seem as obvious, which feels like a superpower to a photographer.

In each interview, I asked creatives to describe what it feels like when they smoke. For some, smoking feels like a widening of scope, tapping into that brainstorming capability related to the default mode network. For others, it leads to hyperfocus and clarity of direction related to the executive attention network. There were some remarkable similarities and some incredibly unique insights offered.

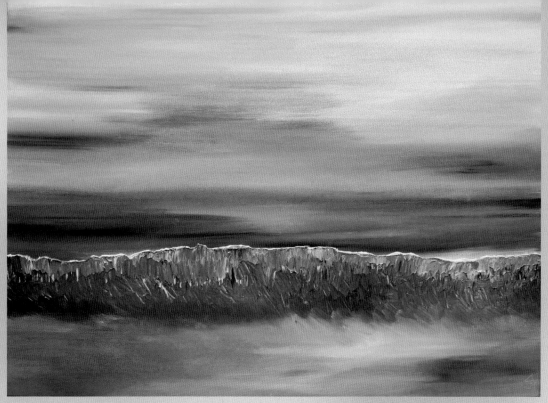

Untitled 130 by Sanjay Patel

"It turns my inner monologue into a quieter conversation. I'm relaxed in my body. I feel my shoulders lower and my spine loosen up. When you're stressed or tense, taking a deep breath helps for a couple of minutes and you think 'OK, that helped.' But then you're right back to where you started. When you smoke, it's like having that deep breath last for a couple of hours."

—Uncle Sexy,
singer-songwriter

"Weed clears other energy from contaminating your creation so the creation can be perfect and in the moment. You want a true expression for what your soul needs without clutter from any other influences. Cannabis brings me back to the moment."

—Trisha Smith,
musician and performer

"We live in such a world of distraction, and once I get distracted, that distraction gets placed into the art. With cannabis, there's a singular voice in your head, which is outside of your own ego even. That's when you can really be focused. There's nothing else pulling you. It's like a state of meditation."

—Sanjay Patel,
painter

"When I'm high, I love the tiny little details. I use a lot of line work, a lot of little creases and folds, I use a lot of pointillism. If you're trying to de-stress, I'm telling the world, get high and do pointillism. It's calming. Self-reflective. You're not going anywhere. Neither is the drawing."

—JBones,
cartoonist

"The biggest part for me is the ability to focus on what I'm doing. As a person with high anxiety and depression, I find it really hard to not worry and think about a million different things. I carry the weight of the day with me, so it's always nice to have that ritual: come home, smoke, and then I'm just zoned in on whatever it is that I want to do. I think that's a big part of functioning better creatively. I'm not overthinking; I'm just focusing on what I'm trying to do."

—Amanda Hosking,
stained-glass artist

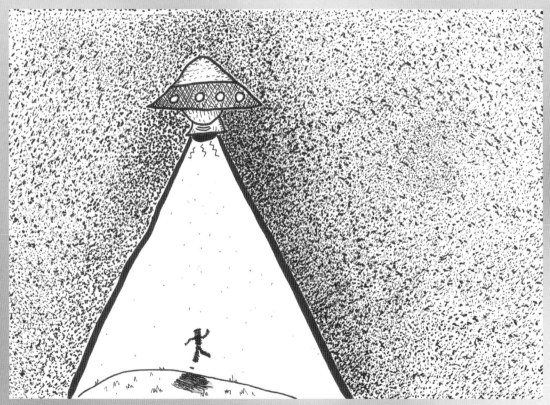

Ink drawing by JBones

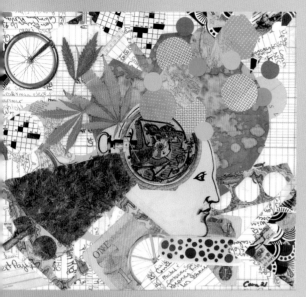

Head Change by Cara Dilluvio

"I definitely do feel something happening. Because I've been doing it for so long, it's not as prominent as it was, but it's still the same kind of cause and effect. I feel like music has more sound to it. If you're looking at something beautiful, there's more sparkle. If you're thinking about something creatively, there's more spark in it when you're high because your brain doesn't have any walls. It's like you let all of the balloons out. Whereas without it, you still have all of those balloons in there, but you're keeping them together. They could be so much cooler looking if they were out there floating around."

—Cara Dilluvio,
    visual artist

"When I'm high, I feel like I see the photos before I take them. When I shoot, I like to get it right in camera. I don't want to rely on all kinds of crazy editing, so I think it helps me really see the shot before I take it. When I'm editing photos, smoking makes it feel more like I can create a story with the image. It brings me on a journey."

—Dariusz Malysa,
    photographer

"I feel like it helps me get more inside of my head, which I think is why some people get anxiety or nervousness or paranoia. It really does put you inside of your body. You really feel everything. It makes food taste better; it makes music sound better. When I paint, it makes the colors more vibrant. It makes me understand how I'm feeling and what I want to see in the art just because I'm more in my own headspace. I'm more conscious of myself and everything that's going on within me."

—Laurel Williams (not her real name),
    visual artist and art teacher

"It helps me get out of my own head. We all tend to have habits or ways of thinking ingrained in our process, and I think smoking [pot] is a good way of shaking things up a little bit and looking at an ingredient differently or a method of preparation differently, or even a flavor combination differently. It gets me out of my own head, so I can access things outside of the box."

—Bruno Wu,
    chef

The Goldilocks Zone

In astronomy, environmental studies, and medical science, you'll frequently hear the term the Goldilocks Zone. Based on everyone's favorite breaking-and-entering parable, the Goldilocks Zone refers to when conditions are ideal for a certain outcome. The porridge isn't too hot, it isn't too cold, it's just right. The earth is in an astronomical Goldilocks Zone—just the right distance from the sun to support a variety of life. The human body's homeostasis relies on Goldilocks Zone conditions too.

The cannabis high, as it relates to creativity, functions within its own Goldilocks Zone. We want to have just enough cannabis in our systems to assist in our creative goals, but not so much that we're rendered a giggling or paranoid pile of mush. Finding the right strain, the right method, and the right dosage are vital for having a successful creative high, but it's not a straightforward process.

Dr. Kaplan explained:

> One of the greatest limitations for someone new to using cannabis is not just navigating the many thousands of different products that are available, but deciding how much to take. There are no use guidelines. You pick up a bottle of Advil, it says, 'Take this many if you weigh this much,' but with cannabis, there's none of that. For different therapeutic indications, whether it's helping with anxiety, helping sleep, treating pain, or some of the more recreational ones, like helping with creativity, what is the optimal dose needed to achieve those effects? And it turns out that actually those effects are only achieved within a somewhat narrow window.

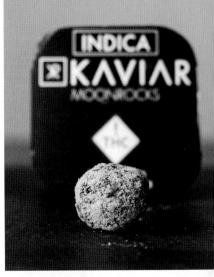

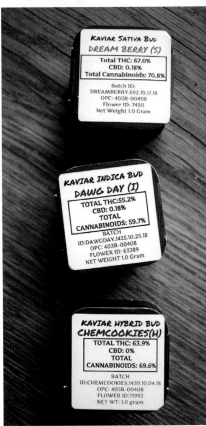

Cannabis products like these Moonrocks by Kaviar have very informative packaging, but they still don't indicate proper dosage.

Think back to the laboratory study of cannabis from the Netherlands mentioned earlier. Participants trended toward heightened creativity with low doses of THC and impaired creativity at higher doses. In that test, the Goldilocks Zone occurred with a lower dose of THC.

Scientists are interested in defining the ideal window of success for cannabis use, but meanwhile, pot smokers are stuck with home experimentation. For those of us who have been imbibing for years, we have a firm grasp of what our cannabis Goldilocks Zone looks like. Newer pot smokers, or people who are just venturing from homegrown pot to designer dispensary products have a lot more work ahead of them in figuring out their ideal dosage and administration methods.

Creative work also requires its own Goldilocks Zone. Many artists rely on just the right conditions to feel focused, energized, and capable of producing their best work. You can't force the creative impulse to appear, but you can set the stage for success. We live in a world of distractions, and for many artists, a ritualized creation process demands carefully curated conditions. Adding cannabis to that equation suggests a special balance of environment and state of mind for creative success.

For the best focus when writing, I know that I need to be alone in a room so I can read my work aloud without feeling self-conscious. I can write some types of content after smoking a hit or two, but if I get too high, I have to wait and come back down a bit. Photography is a looser process. I can edit photos in much more fluid conditions without privacy and have fun doing it even if I'm pretty baked out. My Goldilocks Zone varies from one type of creative pursuit to the next, both in terms of environment and cannabis.

So, what does the creative Goldilocks Zone look like for other artists, and how are they achieving it?

"Part of the inspirational thing about weed comes back to healing ourselves. The only time that I make art that people really relate to on a bigger platform is when I'm in a happy, content place. That doesn't come just from food. It doesn't just come from environment. It doesn't just come from good sex. You can have all of those things, but it doesn't come without marijuana. When I'm high, I create the artwork that everybody loves. Once the paint is there and the canvas is ready and the light is right, and I've had enough to smoke and eat—once all of that happens, the paintings just fly out of me."

—Sanjay Patel,
painter

"When I'm high, I feel like I should be doing something. I get that urge where I want to be productive or trying to progress as a human. I like to smoke and then hop on the CTA [Chicago Transit Authority] and go into the loop and walk around for a couple of hours. Just experience what's going on. See the world. If you put on music and go by yourself it becomes more of a journey. That's when my best work is created. It takes away all the other noise. You get to be with yourself."

—Dariusz Malysa,
photographer

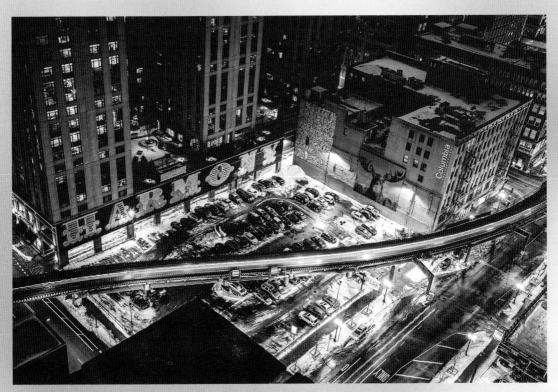

Arteries by Dariusz Malysa

"I'm always listening to music. It makes me anxious to sit in silence, so I will start with some music, and then I'll smoke and make my art. I prefer smoking before I get started, rather than doing it throughout. I want to make sure that I get into the right headspace so I'm not getting so high that I can't focus, because I feel like that definitely can happen too."

—Laurel Williams (not her real name),
visual artist and art teacher

"It usually starts with a base; all my big pieces start with a map or some sort of weird schematic for a machine. If I find a really cool base, that gets me started, and a lot of times it's just finding the perfect elements. I'm constantly picking up stuff. Then, before I start working, instead of just hitting the bong or smoking a joint, I might eat an edible and know that I'm good and I won't have to keep stopping to get higher as I go."

—Cara Dilluvio,
visual artist

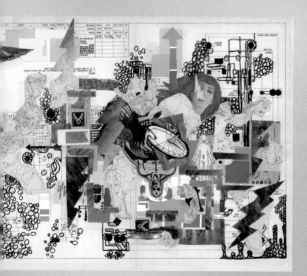

Shocking by Cara Dilluvio

"Cannabis heightens my senses in tasting and experiencing food, and I feel like it also opens my mind to new ideas of food and new ways of experiencing food, so I absolutely believe in the connection between the two. If I'm trying a new recipe out, I'll roll myself a joint and smoke half of it. Then I'll tackle the dish, smoke the other half of the joint, and then I'll taste what I made. If I'm trying to sit down and come up with menu ideas for a client, I'll sit down with a cup of coffee and a small bowl and my notes, and I just focus on that."

—Bruno Wu,
chef

"I've always found it a little bit more helpful to work when high if I don't have a particular set of goals when I'm working, where I'm just kind of screwing around like, 'Alright, let me see if there's something creative that comes to the table' and playing around with that.

I'd never want to do it when I have to achieve something particular. It's definitely more for creative experimentation, when it's a bit more like you're improvising. You're playing jazz, versus needing to sit at the concert and play something more formal."

—Edward Marcus (not his real name),
photographer

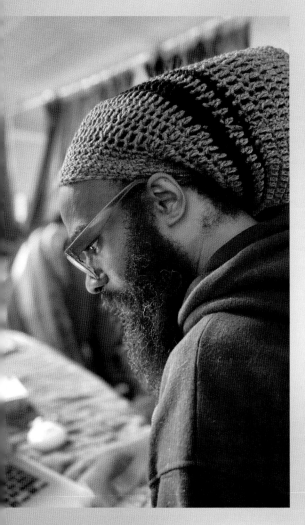

"I smoke, I make my yerba mate, I burn palo santo, I turn on music, and then I write. So cannabis is the first step, and usually cannabis continues on throughout writing, but it always starts off the whole creative process. It gets my mind in the right space to be able to think."

—Gary Wingfield Jr.,
poet

Burning herbs and natty dreads,
kindness serves and happiness spreads.
Each of these is me.
Worldly words and optimistic dunes,
hordes of birds and mystic runes.
Each of these is me.
End each day with gratitude,
it helps my total attitude.
I stay away from platitude,
it helps to watch my latitude.
So that I always stay afloat,
as if in fact I were a boat,
in this wooded wilderness,
away from footprints and foolishness.

—Gary Wingfield Jr.

"First, I'll smoke, make some garbage doodles, just something to get the brain moving, then maybe try to seek inspiration from life: what you're seeing, how you're feeling, how is it outside, what music are you listening to?"

—JBones,
cartoonist

"When it's time to buckle down, I have my little ritual: I take a record, I put it on, I break up the weed on the record sleeve, and I roll it, and then I sit there and I smoke, and then afterwards I just write and it flows so much better."

—Uncle Sexy,
singer-songwriter

Some of the creatives I spoke to can smoke three grams in a bong before working; others prefer the **microdosing** approach to maintain a consistent buzz level. So why is there such a broad level of fluctuation in the types of highs we experience? Some of it has to do with the strain and method of imbibing, but the most significant factor seems to be our body chemistry.

I remember a puff session in college where five of us piled into my closet and passed around a **bowl**. Some of us hit the pipe multiple times without a problem and kept our wits about us. One kid, who'd never smoked with us before, started acting wild a few minutes after his first hit. He claimed his belt was a snake trying to smother him. I can't explain why his body interacted so erratically with pot, but it just goes to show that we are each totally different in our physiological and psychological responses. I've seen inexperienced smokers overdo it and vomit. I've seen some get intensely paranoid and lock themselves in bathrooms. Some people smoke all day, every day, for life and live as productive members of society. Others know that for them, pot is an "only on the weekends" kind of thing for when responsibility is out of the way.

Neuroscientists believe that our responses to cannabis are affected by our age, our experience level, any pharmaceuticals we might be taking, our diet, and even our natural hormone levels. Finding the right strains, methods, quantity, frequency, and environment are all key to developing our own creative Goldilocks Zone, but until research advances a bit more, we're on our own to find what works.

The Top-Down Approach

You can, and many of us will, walk into a dispensary and ask for recommendations for the best energetic high or the best painkilling strain. Many cannabis brands perform independent research to determine which strains have what effects. But knowing what we know about biochemistry and the Goldilocks Zone, just because it says "energetic, creative, happy" on the side of a bottle or on an online strain profile doesn't necessarily make it so.

When developing drugs to treat a specific ailment, laboratory scientists usually synthesize a formula first, then test it on animals, and eventually test it on humans. It's a bottom-up approach. Cannabis presents a unique opportunity for scientists: a chance to utilize existing knowledge and usage patterns in real-world applications and bring them into the lab to better understand what exactly is happening within the body. It's the top-down approach,

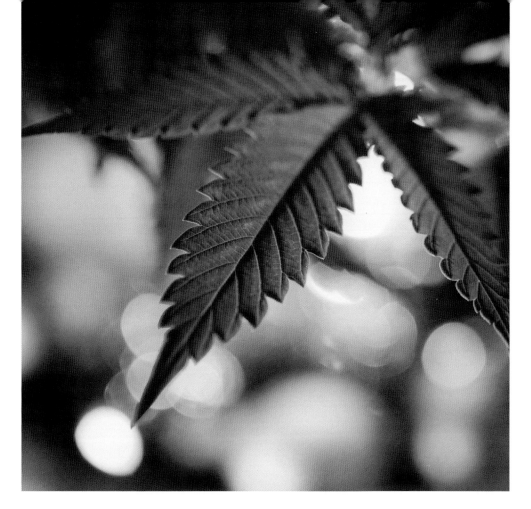

and it means that we're not starting from scratch. We have centuries of historical cannabis use and an enormous wealth of individual experiences, like the interviews in this book, to help shape our understanding of cannabis.

In his lab work, Dr. Kaplan, fueled by anecdotal evidence of children whose epilepsy was helped with cannabis, seeks to understand how exactly it works and how to make it even more effective. The top-down approach.

Many cannabis enthusiasts start experimenting with pot because it's the social thing to do. Whether we find it in high school, college, at a concert, or at a party, it often begins as a communal activity. Then, over time, many start to discover that cannabis can have positive, productive effects in our lives, and our usage shifts. For many of us, that shift is general, occurring with maturation, but some cannabis enthusiasts can pinpoint the exact moment when they began on their own therapeutic and creative path with pot.

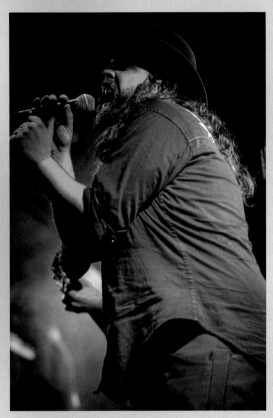

Uncle Sexy performs on stage

"There wasn't necessarily a lightning bolt moment or anything, but I think that it just came with maturity. You get to a point, I think maybe it was towards the end of high school, when you realize that some people are only gonna do this in high school for the party aspect. I do remember I was talking to a friend once and she said, 'Oh man, we're not gonna smoke this forever' or something like that, and I'm like, 'Wait, I think I am…. I find that it helps me.' And she responded, 'Oh no, when I get older, I'm not going to…' And that was kind of when I realized people see this as a different thing than what I view it as, and that was when it became less about fun and more about this is what I like to do, to relax and to expand my brain a little bit."

—Nikki Barber,
   multidisciplinary artist

"In school, I mostly used cannabis as a way to relax in the evening, but once I got out on my own and was able to purchase it easier, it really helped me to expand my creativity. When I was going through school, I was constantly making art for school, and I had a hard time trying to keep that creativity up, so I wish that I would have thought about it as a tool growing up rather than just a recreational thing."

—Laurel Williams (not her real name),
   visual artist and art teacher

"My thoughts were always a little bit chaotic as a kid. I would try to write songs, and it would just be like 10,001 thoughts all jammed into one song, and I could never nail it down. I started smoking a lot more when I was on the road with a band, and I think that really helped me reel everything in. It helps me keep my train of thought going pretty well, and it seems to give me ideas too. I also think it's got a lot to do with altering your perspective. You can appreciate the little things more."

—Uncle Sexy,
   singer-songwriter

"In Mexico, there was this taboo about marijuana. I thought if I smoked, it would make me really stupid or throw my life in the garbage. When I was in Spain, it was very different. It was a more mature way of using cannabis, so people were more free about it. My mind started to change. Then, when I moved to Turks and Caicos, most of my friends would smoke it. After work, we would roll a joint and then start to talk about food and about life. We were connecting a lot and coming up with new ideas."

—Kael Mendoza,
chef

"As Rastas, we are taught to look to the herb for understanding and enlightenment. Although it is not a stipulation, it aids in meditation and reasoning. Rasta, cannabis, and reggae all came to me at the same time. As I smoked, I heard Bob [Marley], I began to grow my hair out. Rasta gave me the match to light the fire of creativity; cannabis was definitely the kindling. As my hair grew, my tolerance did, and so did my blackness. Personal peace, love, and prosperity; those are the Rasta mantras I live by. Cannabis allows me to explore these things without fear of anything. No metaphysical fear, only curiosity, leading me to signs and symbols. Rasta teaches you not to be afraid, ganja is the proof."

—Gary Wingfield Jr,
poet

"When I moved to California, I gained a better general knowledge of what I was smoking. I got my medical card, and it was a different world of information, different products, and different methods of ingestion. That was really cool. Having the knowledge of what exactly I was smoking or vaping helped with adjusting and learning to use different strains to get the desired effect of what I needed it for at the time."

—Bruno Wu,
chef

"I remember the first time that I actually saw light—really, truly saw it and understood it. I was baked out of my mind. As photographers, it usually takes us a while when working with the camera to be able to see where the light is coming from and where it's going, and how it falls off, and how it bounces. I was leaning over a friend's counter and was really stoned, and I remember seeing the light bounce off someone's lip, and then I saw the reflection of the light on the other lip, and it all clicked for me. I don't know if it's something that I would have noticed normally. It vibrates your attention and flexes what you're focusing on. I remember seeing that and going, 'Oh, that's it.' The math of it made sense all of a sudden. It completely changed my ability to see everything from then on out. I could see the physicality of light."

—Edward Marcus (not his real name),
photographer

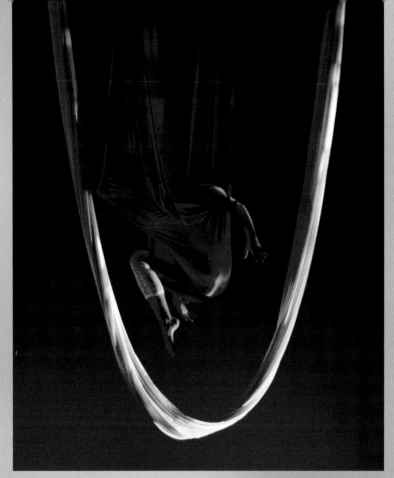

Lighting designer Cassius Wright prefers to select colors after smoking.

"When I was first learning how to do lighting design in college and would have to pick color for a show, I had a lot of anxiety about it because I was working with people who had much more experience. My professor always picked colors so beautifully, and I asked him how he did it. He said that he picked color when he was so tired he couldn't think straight. He would do it as fast as he could, and always completely exhausted. I thought, 'Alright, well, how can I put myself in this state to practice picking colors?' I began smoking specifically when I needed to pick lighting design colors, and I have always picked absolutely fantastic colors that way. In the creative process of lighting design, there are very few things that you can't execute more effectively when you're high."

—Cassius Wright,
   lighting and event designer

Outward-In Mentality

For decades, psychologists have studied the extent to which acting out an emotion can manifest it. Some studies have claimed that the act of smiling makes us feel happier. Putting our hands on our hips in a "power pose" can result in a rush of self-confidence and capability. So, the question arises: are we feeling more creative when we're high because we believe cannabis can have that effect? How much have statements from artists over the years influenced the way we feel when stoned?

As Dr. Kaplan explained to me:

> With a drug like cannabis, there's so much inherent bias in people's use. We've known this since the '60s. Some of those early reports coming out of UCLA talked about the critical element of set and setting. If people expect something to work, it's gonna work a lot better than when they don't [expect it to]. So, when you think it's gonna make you feel creative and enhance your artistic ability or musical ability, you're going to subjectively say that it's going to work. We are really powerful drivers of our own brain chemistry. It's that outward-in mentality. If you just start smiling a lot, you're gonna actually feel happier. We have control to some degree over our brain chemistry. The question is whether or not that's working in actuality, in a kind of an unbiased, objective manner. That's a different story, and I think we're just starting to crack that one open. That's why having objective empirical studies is so important to understand this from a scientific perspective.

In his book, *Understanding Marijuana*, Dr. Mitch Earleywine suggests that cannabis and creativity are somewhat of a "chicken-and-egg" dilemma. He references a 1977 study that demonstrated superior cognitive test scores among cannabis users over non-users. Dr. Earleywine questions the efficacy of the testing measures:

> The superior performance of marijuana users may stem, in part, from the nature of the measures. Unlike the tests employed in most studies, these focused on originality and novel thinking rather than speedy processing of information. These data do not, however, mean marijuana smokers are more creative than others. The groups may have differed in originality prior to use.

A 2017 lab study titled "Inspired by Mary Jane? Mechanisms underlying enhanced creativity in cannabis users," concluded that personality differences have a lot to do with perceived creativity. Divergent thinking increased temporarily when experienced smokers got high, but "both perceived and objective differences in sober cannabis users' and non-users' creativity appear to be merely a function of cannabis users' higher levels of openness to experience."

So, does cannabis make us more creative, or is it that creative people are more open to using mind-altering substances and exploring these psychotropic experiences for the sake of art?

Dr. Earleywine thinks it's a little bit of each, saying:

> *While smoking cannabis, people often behave in ways that would change their emotions, even in the absence of the drug. Listening to music, savoring favorite foods, and enjoying other activities stereotypically paired with marijuana consumption may provide some of the euphoria usually attributed to the substance. People may say that marijuana makes them happy, when, in fact, it is the chance to watch TV, have sex, or walk in the woods that actually improves their moods. In addition, some cannabis effects may stem from expectations rather than pharmacology. People may expect a drug to make them happy and may end up feeling happy simply as a result of the expectation.*

When we condition ourselves to come home from work and smoke to relax, we start that relaxation process through expectation. If we believe it will make us more creative, is it actually having that effect, or are we manifesting our own creativity?

Of the subjects I interviewed, some believed wholeheartedly that cannabis was making them more creative. They see a causal relationship. Others believe it just helps eliminate distractions, negativity, and anything else that gets in the way of the creative process. They believe that, much like curating your physical environment, curating your creative experience with cannabis can open doors you might otherwise walk right by.

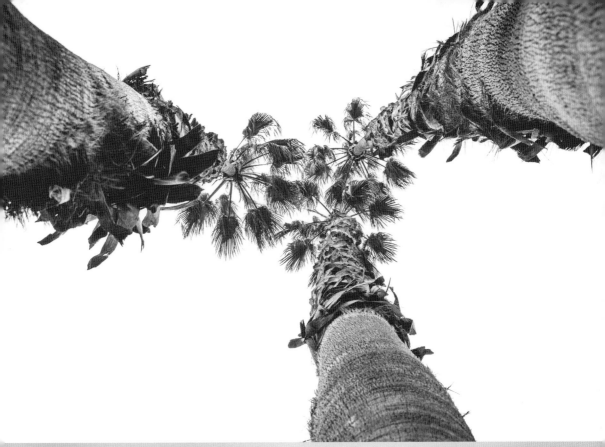

PWA by Dariusz Malysa

"It gives you a different view of beauty. It just opens up a whole different pathway that you wouldn't normally experience. Some people just walk by something and wouldn't even have looked at it twice, but I see it and know that it could be a piece of art."

—Dariusz Malysa,
   photographer

"Cannabis definitely helps me feel creative. When I make commissioned art, it's really hard to get started, so I feel like cannabis gets me the motivation I need. If I'm painting something for myself, sometimes I get to parts where I think I'm done because I don't know what else I could add. Cannabis helps me to get more into my head so that I can think about what else it could use or what else I could do to make it better."

—Laurel Williams (not her real name),
   visual artist and art teacher

"I don't think it's a linear process where you induce cannabis and then something happens; it's just that by including cannabis in the whole process, you let down guards that you normally keep up. Pot dials up something that already exists, it does not bring anything new to your experience. Having that [high] perspective on whatever the topic is may support the creative process; therefore, you have more perspectives and also more access to things you would normally shy away from."

—Juerg "Fed" Federer,
chef, writer, and creativity consultant

"Cannabis definitely helps me access creativity more easily. When I smoke weed and I listen to a song, the weed just helps make it way more colorful and way more imaginative. I feel like I'm transported somewhere else, like I'm in some sort of setting that fits with the song perfectly."

—Anna Pollock,
visual artist

"When you're smoking weed, you have no hindrances, and you don't doubt yourself. Every time you step back to look at your art, every time you pause for a moment, you're asking, 'Was that good enough? Was that the right choice?' Smoking puts you in the moment, and if you are right in the moment you don't need to ask those questions."

—Trisha Smith,
musician and performer

"When I haven't smoked, my scope is very wide. I'll get distracted easily. When I'm smoking cannabis and I'm drawing, I'm just worrying about the art, which really isn't a worry at all. I'm just so honed in. I'm in way less pain. I feel more creative. I just feel like I'm a better person because of it. I'm drawing my best work."

—JBones,
cartoonist

"Not only does it help me organize my thoughts, but it helps me slow things down in general so I can appreciate one thing at a time instead of thinking about 47 things at once. Sometimes I'll write a million thoughts down or whatever I can get, but when I smoke, I'm able to think through it and say, 'OK, this is the thought that matters.' If I were to try to take all of those thoughts and write them all out into a song, it wouldn't work. But if I was stoned, I would be able to decide which lines worked and how to put them together."

—Uncle Sexy,
singer-songwriter

"I've definitely had some creative break-throughs with it. We tend to put so many different rules on ourselves that don't necessarily need to be there in our day-to-day workflow and our formal structure of approach. It definitely lets you either ignore those rules or forget them. It lets you connect point A to point C while being able to bypass B. Or maybe you jump back and forth around and do things totally out of order, and it invites a totally different, new way to do things. A removal of structure sometimes allows you to get out of your own way."

—Edward Marcus (not his real name),
 photographer

"I feel it unlocks what's already there. That's the best way to describe it. It clears my third eye and allows me to see what's already there that I may not have been able to see. It's like a conduit. It brings all of my emotions to the forefront to be able to release but also to be able to recharge at the same time by writing."

—Gary Wingfield Jr,
 poet

"It helps me come up with different ways to solve the same problem. If I need to fix something or need to do something I've never done before, instead of stressing and wondering, 'How am I gonna do this perfectly? Am I gonna get this right?' It's more like, 'Meh. I'll figure it out.' It takes the perfectionism out of it and I enjoy it more."

—Amanda Hosking,
 stained-glass artist

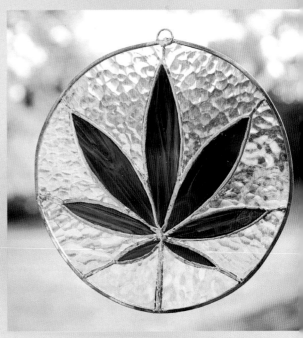

Stained glass by Amanda Hosking

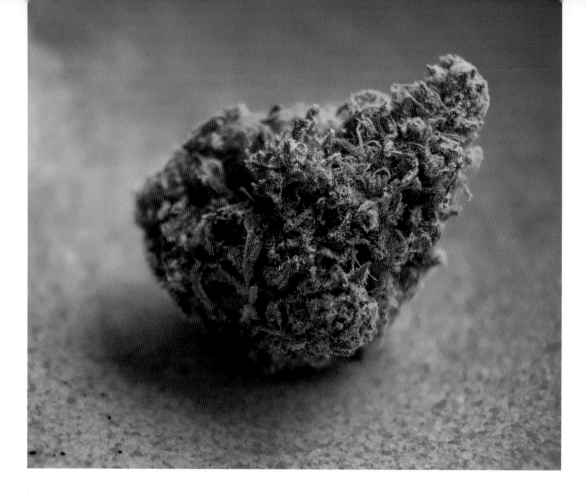

Drawing Conclusions About Cannabis and the Brain

Unsurprisingly, the deeply varied experiences of cannabis users and difficulties in studying those experiences in a regimented laboratory setting, leads to more questions than answers.

Here's what we know: cannabis interacts with a naturally occurring system in the brain to interrupt a variety of psychological and biological processes. Some of those interruptions can be beneficial; some can be detrimental. Just how much interference we experience is based on several factors, most significantly our body chemistry.

Regardless of what laboratory studies turn up in the future, cannabis enthusiasts will continue on as generations have before them. By experimenting with dosage, strain, environment, and other factors, we can effectively curate our experience. We can call forth creativity as long as we hit that magic Goldilocks Zone and figure out how to stay there.

CHAPTER 4

UNDERSTANDING THE PLANT

Cannabis is a magical plant. It can treat a variety of ailments, relieve pain, ease anxiety, cause laughter, inspire introspection, and make you relax. You can smoke it. You can vaporize it. You can eat it. You can absorb it through your skin. You can make paper, clothing, rope, and sailcloth from its fibers. As acceptance of cannabis becomes more pervasive, new methods of ingestion and new therapeutic uses are developed every day. Cannabis—this magical plant once forced underground by propaganda and prohibition—is coming back with a vengeance, and its possibilities seem endless. But how much do we, as consumers, actually understand what it is and what it does?

The Psychoactive Properties of Pot

Cannabis contains hundreds of chemical compounds, each with their own effects and functions. Some of these compounds, such as chlorophyll, omega fatty acids, and lipids, are common among many species of plants. Other compounds are more unique to cannabis. When talking about the psychoactive properties of pot, we're primarily addressing *cannabinoids* and *terpenes*.

Cannabinoids

As we've learned, cannabinoids interact with our body's endocannabinoid system to synthesize the psychoactive and therapeutic effects we know and love. The cannabinoid we talk about most frequently is THC, but it's just one of many cannabinoids found in pot.

Here are a few of the key cannabinoids we are likely to encounter in our lives as cannabis enthusiasts:

Tetrahydrocannabinol (THC)

Widely regarded as the most important component in catching a buzz or feeling high, THC is released most effectively when heated, by smoking, vaping, or when cooked into butter or ghee. Most often, when you read or hear about THC, it's in reference to delta-9-tetrahydrocannabinol. There is a very similar compound called delta-8-tetrahydrocannabinol that can be found in cannabis and in hemp. In most circumstances, delta-8 offers more mild psychoactive effects. For the purposes of this book, we focus on delta-9 THC.

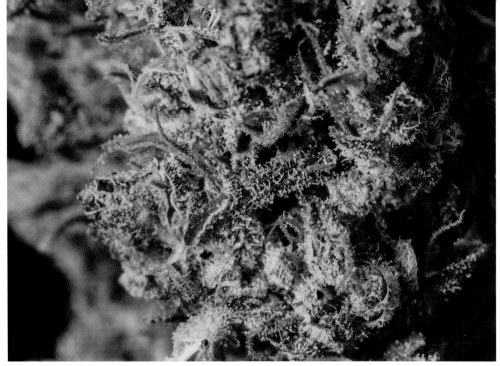

Treasure Island is a strain with a 15:1 CBD to THC ratio, so while you may not feel high after smoking it, you will feel pleasantly relaxed.

Cannabidiol (CBD)

CBD is increasingly in the spotlight because of its positive effects for relaxation, pain relief, anxiety and inflammation reduction, and treatment of seizures. CBD doesn't make you feel high, but it can make you feel very chill. CBD can also help reduce some of the potentially negative psychoactive effects of THC like panic and anxiety.

Cannabinol (CBN)

With mild psychoactive effects, CBN is an increasingly popular cannabinoid for therapeutic purposes in treating epilepsy, cancer, nausea, and glaucoma. CBN is a natural byproduct that can occur when THC breaks down with age or exposure to the elements, but it is also found in strains grown outdoors.

Cannabigerol (CBG)

Another non-psychoactive ingredient, CBG helps with blood pressure, sleep, and inflammation. It isn't as ubiquitous as other cannabinoids in many strains on the market, but it's gaining popularity.

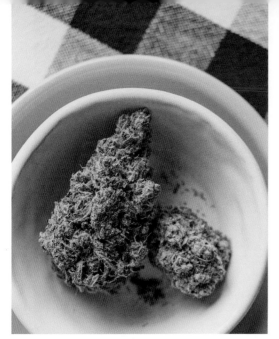
Cherrygasm

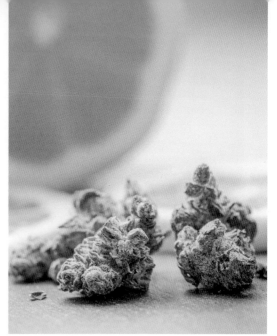
Sour Amnesia

Terpenes

When you talk to a true enthusiast about cannabis, they'll often mention terpenes. Terpenes are the natural oils in cannabis that are largely responsible for aroma and flavor, so when you come across a skunky strain, a citrusy strain, or a cheesy strain, you have terpenes to thank. Many people associate terpenes specifically with cannabis, but terpenes are found in a variety of plants and common fragrances. Each cannabis strain can include multiple terpenes, which helps add to the richness of aroma and effect.

Here are just a few of the terpenes you'll commonly encounter on a trip to the dispensary:

Limonene
Limonene smells how it sounds: citrusy and delightful. It's believed to elevate mood and relieve stress and can also be found in the rind of citrus fruits. Popular limonene strains include Wedding Cake, MAC, Purple Hindu Kush, and Berry White.

Linalool
Imagine walking through a field of fresh lavender. That relaxing and calming sensation you might experience is thanks to linalool. Strains with linalool frequently have a floral scent. Smoke a linalool strain, like Do-Si-Dos or Kosher Kush, and you may feel less anxious.

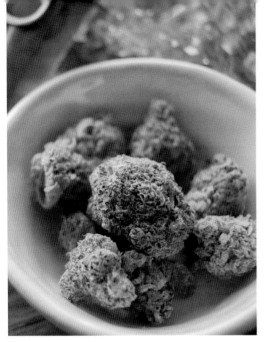
Lavender Jones

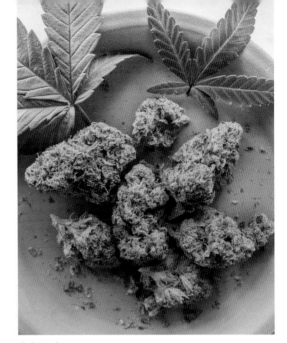
OG Kush

Pinene

Pinene is perhaps the most frequently found terpene in nature. It also smells how it sounds: piney and refreshing. Pinene exists naturally in coniferous plants, basil, and rosemary, and is appreciated for its uplifting effects. Popular pinene strains include Blue Dream, Cannatonic, Grape Ape, and Cotton Candy Kush.

Humulene

Bring on the earthy strains like Sour Diesel, White Widow, and Girl Scout Cookies. Cannabis that's high in humulene is often referred to as "dank." Humulene is also found in cloves and hops. It's believed to have anti-inflammatory properties.

Caryophyllene

The super spicy terpene caryophyllene appears in strains like OG Kush, Chem Dog, Sour Diesel, and Bubba Kush. It also naturally occurs in black pepper, cinnamon, and cloves. Caryophyllene is believed to interact with CB2 receptors, so it's commonly used in topical products for anti-inflammatory purposes. It also has antidepressant properties.

Myrcene

Delightfully earthy, myrcene is known for its calming properties. It's found in lemongrass, hops, and mango, but in the cannabis world, it's frequently found in Blue Dream, and White Widow.

How Cannabis Compounds Work Together

If you've done your cannabis research, you may have come across something called The Entourage Effect. Recently, researchers have begun to realize that the way our bodies and minds react to cannabis isn't all that straightforward or predictable. We used to believe that pot's effects were associated entirely with a plant's taxonomy. Indica would put you down, and sativa would lift you up. The indica vs. sativa taxonomy discussion is fairly complex and is still a source of conflict among cannabis researchers (more on this later), but recent theories suggest that cannabis's effects occur due to the overall collection of chemical compounds found in the strains we ingest. In essence, it's not just the DJ who brings the party, you need the whole entourage.

A strain's specific balance of cannabinoids and terpenes mixed with our individual biochemistry are responsible for us feeling creative or tired or relaxed or energetic. That's why it can be so complicated to find our personal Goldilocks Zone. One dispensary's Gorilla Glue might inspire productivity, while another dispensary's Gorilla Glue might lock you in a couch for the next four to six hours. I might smoke the same strain as my husband, and he's dancing around while I stare into space, lost in thought.

Many cannabis companies have embraced the entourage effect because it helps them market products like vape pens with targeted outcomes: use this pen for a productive high or use that one for relaxation. But for now, in the absence of standardization and extensive lab testing, those promises seem to be mostly marketing. Our sample list of terpenes includes plenty of expected responses, but since you're never smoking just one terpene, lots of other cannabinoids and chemical elements come into play.

What's in a Name: Sativa, Indica, Ruderalis, and Hemp

Discussions of sativa and indica and the myth those terms have come to represent is one of the quickest ways to get peace-loving, hippy-minded potheads all in a tizzy. Here's where the craziness began…

In 1753, Carl Linnaeus, a Swedish botanist, formally named cannabis plants Cannabis Sativa. Then in 1785, Jean-Baptiste Lamarck, a French biologist, came along and decided

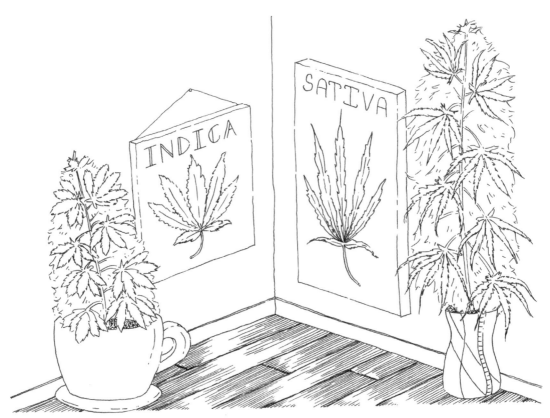

Indica and sativa may look different, but genetically they're fairly identical. (Illustration by John McAmis)

that Cannabis Indica was a separate species because it looked different. Differences in plant height, bushiness, leaf thickness, and overall appearance made Lamarck feel certain that there were two entirely separate species of cannabis. (Lamarck was also under the impression that physical changes in our bodies occurring over the course of our lifetimes are passed on to our children, but that's a whole other weird giraffe-based theory that was dispensed with in favor of Darwinian evolution.)

Like many things we believed in the 18th century, the sativa and indica titles stuck, and in the 1930s a Russian botanist named Dmitrij Janischewsky added a third cannabis "species," ruderalis, into the mix. Ruderalis doesn't vary much from sativa or indica plants in any physical way, but it does tend to be significantly less psychoactive with fewer and smaller buds, much lower in THC.

Over the past few centuries, the term *hemp* has been used to describe cannabis grown as a crop for fibers and oils. It is legally classified in the United States as a cannabis plant

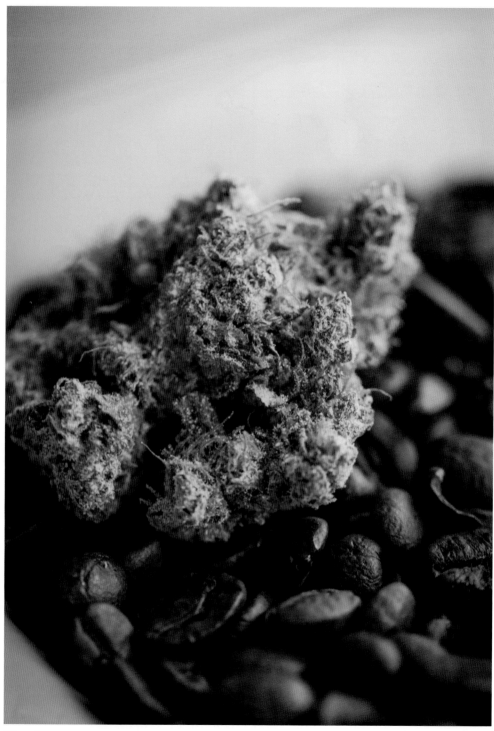

Chocolope

CANNABIS FOR CREATIVES

containing 0.3% or less THC. Because it lacks psychoactive capabilities, many governments are willing to explore hemp as an agricultural product even while classifying psychoactive cannabis as an illegal drug. Hemp can be used as a source of dietary protein as well as a crop for producing paper, clothing, biodegradable plastics, and more, but as one of my high-school friends learned the hard way with a hemp bracelet and a moment of desperation, it's not worth smoking.

Over the past 250-ish years, sativa, indica, ruderalis, and hemp have been treated as distinct species with completely different physical attributes (which is mostly accurate), psychoactive attributes (maybe somewhat accurate), and genetic attributes (quite inaccurate). We're just starting to see the error of our ways.

Sativa: What We Know

Sativa strains are generally identified as being tall and lanky. Branches are spread out across a large physical area. It's not uncommon to see sativa plants reach five feet or more in height. Sativa leaves have long, thin fingers set far apart, and they are generally a light green color. Sativa buds are more spindly and loose.

Some of the first sativa strains identified were found in tropical and subtropical regions. These areas have a long growing season and are prone to more prolonged heat and high humidity. Those environmental conditions led to the proliferation of enormous plants, which allowed plenty of airflow between leaves, branches, and buds. Plants that demonstrated better air circulation were more likely to survive through threats of mold and mildew to the flowering stage. Over time, these phenotypic, or observable physical traits, became the defining characteristics of "sativa" plants.

Indica: What We Know

Indica strains are usually identified as being short and compact. Branching is tight and plants remain relatively short and bushy. Indica leaves are characterized as having shorter and wider fingers that sometimes overlap. They also tend to be darker in color. Buds are dense and fat.

The first indica strains were identified in the mountainous Hindu Kush region in Central Asia. Because they developed and proliferated in a region known for more erratic weather, higher altitudes, extreme gusts of wind, and a shorter growing season, the most biologically successful indica strains were hearty and short. They could better withstand wind by remaining closer to the ground, which also allowed them to save their resources for bigger, heartier buds to help propagate the species. More robust leaves meant they could absorb all of the available sunlight even during unpredictable weather. Potential cold snaps and snow were far easier to survive for a plant with the phenotypic traits of a compact "indica."

Sativa and Indica: Where Things Get Tricky

For as long as humans have known about the many benefits of cannabis, we've been transporting seeds around the globe. Some plants don't survive very well outside their ideal growing zone. Take a look at any nursery catalog, and you'll realize how much work you have cut out for you if you attempt growing a native Floridian species outdoors in Montana. (Spoiler alert: your orange tree is going to die in 10 feet of snow.) But cannabis is called

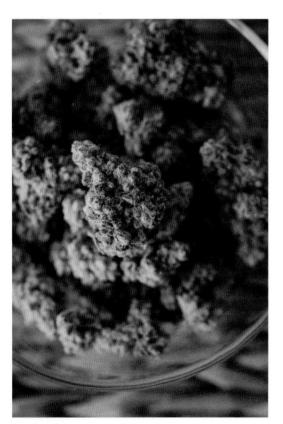

Tom Ford

"weed" for a reason. It will grow practically anywhere you put it. So, when explorers, traders, and hippies traverse continents dropping seeds along the way, they're helping one of earth's heartiest plants proliferate in new climates and under new conditions. Pot adapts to new environments fairly well, and over generations specimens will look very different from the original plant that provided the initial seeds.

Another complicating factor is that cannabis is capable of crossbreeding with any other plant in the cannabis family. Instead of ending up with infertile offspring like the mules produced by donkeys and horses, a pot plant with indica traits can breed with a sativa-traited plant and result in a fantastically fertile specimen. Both sativa and indica can breed with ruderalis or hemp, so nothing stays pure for very long.

In essence, all the cannabis plants on this earth, from wild growing ditch-weed to the specimens you find in commercial grow rooms, have been interfered with by humans over the course of thousands of years. We would know a lot more about cannabis if we had the original plant to reference, but we don't. Humans have been messing around with pot for far longer than we've been studying botany on a scientific level. Pure, unadulterated cannabis just doesn't exist anymore. As a result, no indicas can be truly 100% indica, and no sativas can be 100% purely sativa.

What About Landrace Strains?

A **landrace strain** is a variety of pot that has grown with relatively limited interference over a long period of time in a particular environment. They are some of the purest varieties of cannabis that we know of. They're far less common now than they were even in the 1960s, thanks to human intervention and crossbreeding, and in some circles these strains are like the holy grail. If you're a cannabis connoisseur, you know the unbridled excitement of getting your hands on a landrace strain. In high school, I had a friend whose uncle sent him some bluish-purple nuggets from Hawaii, and we celebrated for a week.

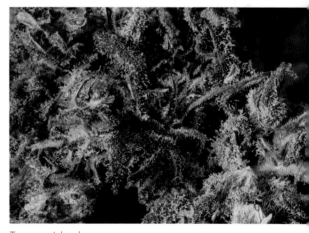

Treasure Island

Popular varieties of landrace strains include: Acapulco Gold (Mexico), Durban Poison (Africa), Lambs Bread (Jamaica), Panama Red (South America), Colombian Gold (South America), Punto Rojo (South America), Thai (Asia), Chocolate Thai (Asia), Afghani (Afghanistan), Hindu Kush (Afghanistan), Maui Wowie (Hawaii), Kona Gold (Hawaii), and many more.

Each of these strains grew with minimal interference in relative isolation for generations. Attributes like stickiness, bud density, aroma, and flavor helped to attract pollinators and animals that would help the plants successfully proliferate. Qualities like branching, size, leaf shape, and growth rate favored specimens most capable of surviving in each individual climate and environment. As a result, they adapted through a similar evolutionary process to Darwin's finches, ultimately becoming the best possible specimens for surviving in their particular environments with the resources available. They are very different from each other physically and psychoactively because of this adaptation, but they likely all originated from a shared lineage.

While many of these strains are typically labeled as sativas or indicas because of their physical characteristics, recent scientific studies performed on a genetic level show that these classifications aren't accurate predictors when it comes to psychoactive effects or even the origin of each specimen.

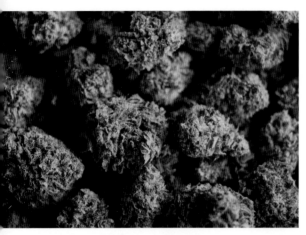

Grape Crush

Exploring Cannabis's Genome

The Cannabis Genomics Research Initiative (CGRI), based in Boulder, Colorado, has spent the past few years working toward a variety of scientific goals, including providing insight about the ways different strains of cannabis are genetically related to each other. Their research could potentially end the sativa vs. indica debate once and for all.

I spoke with Ezra Huscher, one of CGRI's contributing scientists, about their work to help clarify the classification of cannabis. He explained that in an effort to map cannabis's genome, CGRI has gathered hundreds of specimens from dispensaries, former hemp fields in the American Midwest, and other countries. Using these samples, they're building a phylogenetic tree to determine how current cannabis strains are related and how far back those relationships go.

He explained, "It's the same idea as if you're gonna do a phylogenetic tree of humans and where our species branched off. Further up the branch, you would have apes, chimps would be there, and orangutans, and then you'd go further back, and you eventually get to any species with a backbone, different vertebrates and whatnot. You can look at a phylogenetic tree and see how far back you had the same ancestor."

Through this mapping, Huscher and his colleagues have found that some specimens share obvious grouped lineages. For example, many of the Afghan Kush specimens that they collected from multiple dispensaries were very similar genetically, suggesting that they came from common ancestors. Maui Wowie and Hawaiian (the strain name not the place) were also genetically linked because all strains from the Hawaiian Islands were bred in relative isolation for a very long time. Other strains seemed far more random and individualized in their labeling and genetic background.

When it comes to the titles we assign to strains, Huscher explains that there's no universal system of classification. "It's basically the Wild West out there. People can name strains anything that they want. There's no rhyme or reason to it. Every day, there's probably a dozen new names that people are coming up with in California, in

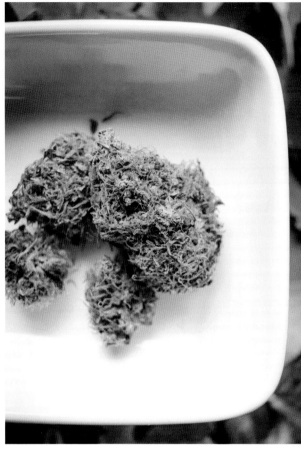

Matanuska Thunderfuck is a wildly named and wildly tasty strain.

Colorado, in these states where the industry is really hopping." Sometimes those titles are based on the parent strains that were involved, but other times names are based on flavor profiles, type of high, or even a famous stoner.

In my early days of smoking, local dealers (much like their contemporary dispensary counterparts) selected strain titles based on what sounded exotic and guaranteed to provide a good time. It was, and still is, deeply related to marketing and sales goals. Because of the limited standardization of genetics from breeder to breeder, dispensaries and freelance cannabis entrepreneurs remain free to name strains anything they want—as anyone who's ever bought Matanuska Thunderfuck or Donkey Dick can attest to.

Ultimately, in mapping cannabis's genome, CGRI hopes to isolate certain genetic qualities, including combinations of terpenes and cannabinoids that will have larger medical implications. In the meantime, they're working through a variety of studies that have so far demonstrated that classifications of indica and sativa are far more arbitrary than your average cannabis enthusiast might realize.

In a follow-up email to our conversation, Huscher reflected:

> *Dispensaries need to put strains into some categories for sales purposes. They are drawing on the historical bifurcation of indicas and sativas, which appear different based on the obvious physical traits. It is my belief, from personal experience and conversations, that not all sativas provide an 'energetic high,' and not all indicas are 'couch-oriented body highs.' They may provide that result more than 50% of the time to justify this generalization somewhat, but certainly not 100% of the time. The complex biochemistry of humans, which differs in every individual, likely leads to a different high. The plant is marvelously complicated and needs much more careful study.*

Growing Like a Weed

Whether or not you imbibe cannabis, growing your own pet pot plant can be a fabulously enriching pastime. While living in Colorado, I took advantage of my legal ability to cultivate my own plant at home and learned so much from my hands-on opportunity about the life cycle and growth stages of pot. If you've never had the chance to experience it for yourself, or if you've never really put any thought into the how and why of cannabis cultivation, here's a quick introduction.

The Basics of Cannabis Anatomy

Cannabis is a *dioecious* plant, meaning that it can be male or female. While female plants are valued for the robust resinous flowers (buds) that contain the bulk of cannabis's psychoactive compounds, male plants are also useful and necessary. Male plants produce the pollen sacs that pollinate female plants and allow future propagation of the species. Fertilized seeds are found in female cannabis buds. While we tend to get annoyed about finding seeds in our expensive buds, they begin the cannabis life cycle.

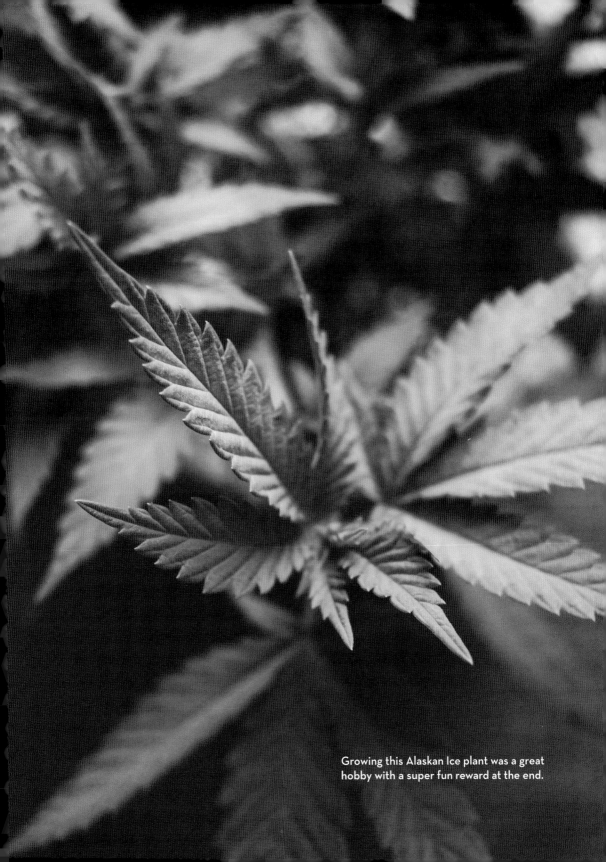

Growing this Alaskan Ice plant was a great
hobby with a super fun reward at the end.

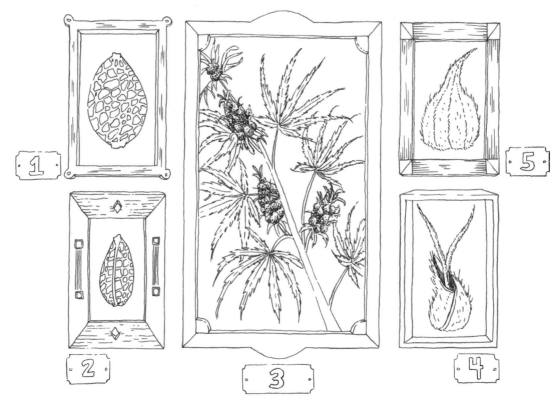

1 & 2: a cannabis seed viewed from the front and side, 3: a mature cannabis plant with fan leaves and buds, 4: stigmas extending from a bract, 5: fully enclosed bract. (Illustration by John McAmis)

Once planted, a pot seed's hard shell opens to reveal a *taproot* (the very first root) and a pair of *cotyledon* leaves. The cotyledons are small, rounded leaves that absorb light to give the plant the initial energy it needs to grow and develop. While leaves grow to pull energy from the sun, roots grow below the soil to gather moisture and nutrients to feed the plant.

Next, a central stalk grows from the base of the cotyledons and forms the physical support system for the plant. Along the stem, you will find nodes, or junction points, between the stem and lateral branches. At first, it may appear that leaves are growing from the stem itself, but early leaves often indicate node sites where future branches will grow and lead to more leaves, and ultimately, flowers.

Fan leaves are what you picture when you think of a pot leaf. They are the larger, multi-pointed, light absorbing leaves. Fan leaves serve a valuable purpose during growth but are generally discarded during harvest because they lack psychoactive resin. Smaller leaves, called *sugar leaves*, are also present, and they tend to be covered in crystals and resin, so they're removed and saved for creating things like hash, kief, edibles, and extracts.

Flowers, or buds, are the fruits of the pot farmer's labor. They can be long and wispy or fat and dense. They can be green, purple, or any color in between. Traditionally, an unmanicured pot plant will produce a primary central bud called the main *cola*, but other branches can produce secondary and tertiary buds as well. Throughout the buds, you'll find *bracts* and *calyxes*. These are small, fuzzy-looking, teardrop-shaped structures that contain the female reproductive components. Bracts and calyxes have a high cannabinoid and terpene concentration. *Stigmas* are the thin red hairs that extend from the buds and catch the pollen from male cannabis plants for fertilization.

Trichomes are often the star of the show when it comes to the cannabis flower. To the naked eye, they appear as white hairs or crystals, but under a microscope they actually look like a sea of tiny round-topped mushrooms. Trichomes are what make pot buds sticky and resinous, and they contain a multitude of cannabinoids and terpenes.

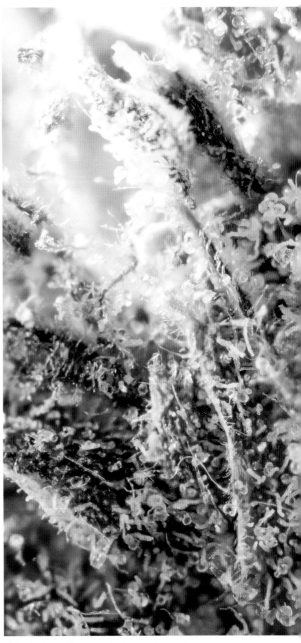

This strain, called Nerds, is resplendent with stigmas and trichomes.

Stages of Growth

After the germination stage (from seed to taproot and cotyledons) and seedling stage (a baby pot plant with a couple of early fan leaves), cannabis plants experience two primary stages of growth: the vegetative stage and the flowering stage.

In the vegetative stage, the structural elements of the plant form. Stems grow tall, branches extend from the stem, and fan leaves grow to harness light. Nutrition and maximized sunlight are especially important. The bigger and healthier the plant, the more capable it will be to grow robust flowers later.

In the natural seasonal cycle of sunlight, the flowering stage is typically triggered by increasing hours of uninterrupted darkness as summer turns to fall. This is the case for both indica and sativa-appearing plants. (Ruderalis specimens function a little differently. They are *autoflowering*, which means they will automatically begin to flower after a certain number of days, regardless of light cycle.) The plants take light changes as a cue that winter is coming, and rather than continuing to grow big and tall, all energy is diverted into developing flowers to help future generations. Many cannabis growers will also cut some of the fan leaves at this stage to help the plant conserve energy and focus all resources on bud development. This is also when a plant will begin to show male or female reproductive structures.

Over a period of weeks (the duration varies greatly by strain), buds grow and develop. Buds in the early stages of growth appear very light green, but over time they ripen, red hairs appear, and they take on the typical appearance we're used to seeing in photographs.

1: A germinated cannabis seed opens, 2: the initial taproot extends into the soil, 3: the seedling breaks the surface of the soil, 4: the cotyledons unfold to capture sunlight, 5: the central stalk grows early fan leaves, 6: the plant grows tall and hearty during the vegetative stage, 7: early buds begin to form during the beginning of the flowering stage, 8: robust buds ripen as harvest approaches. (Illustration by John McAmis)

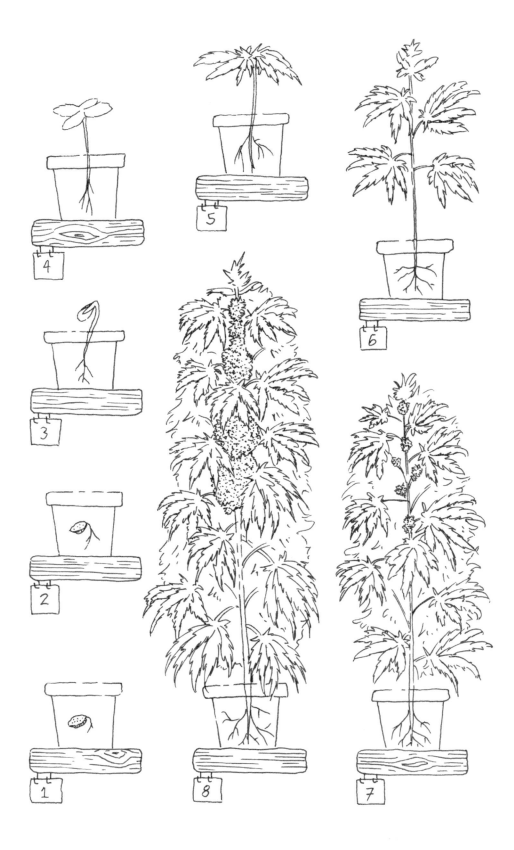

Harvesting Buds

When the buds are fully developed, the plants are ready to be harvested and dried. Growers cut plants at the base of the stem, remove fan leaves, and hang the plants so excess moisture can evaporate. Soon the buds will be ready for trimming.

The trimming process involves removing all excess vegetation. For a cleaner smoke (less throat burn and a better taste), it's best if sugar leaves are fully removed. I've worked as a trimmer for a few growers over the years, and my fine motor skills and attention to detail have really come in handy for manicuring beautiful buds. It can be a very meditative activity. As long as you're not talking about hand-cutting warehouses full of pot, this is one of the most fun parts.

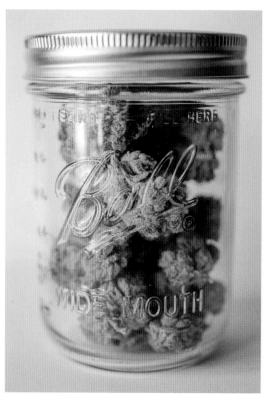

Curing and storing cannabis in airtight containers helps control the dehydration process and enriches flavor and scent.

Once trimmed, buds are further dried and cured in airtight containers to help bring out the natural flavors and aromas. This process is a delicate balance with a goal of between 50–60% relative humidity. It's not all that fun to smoke pot that hasn't been allowed to dry fully or that has been overdried. Cultivation is an art in and of itself.

Indoor vs. Outdoor Growing

Outdoor grows are the traditional and time-honored method. If you're lucky enough to grow in a sunny location with frequent rain, like Humboldt County in California, the growing process will require much less intervention. In the right environment, outdoor plants can become impressive giants—sometimes six or more feet tall. But with the ease of outdoor cultivation also comes the threat of pests, unexpected weather patterns, and the inability to control pollination.

Indoor grows used to be the best method for keeping a pot grow secret, but even in legalized locations they provide an element of control that many farmers prefer. Indoor grows allow precise administration of light, nutrition, and water.

Advanced Growing

These days, cannabis cultivation is often an exact science. Lighting equipment targets the ideal wavelengths for certain phases of growth. Plants can be grown in soil, water, or air. Breeding is controlled for flavor, effect, and look. Modern manicuring techniques like using screens create an even canopy and allow growers to ensure a more robust collection of evenly sized buds for commercial distribution.

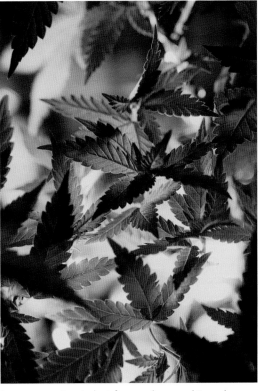

I grew my pet pot plant from a clone, and it made the whole process easier.

In discussions of pot cultivation, you'll often hear about growing from clones rather than from seeds. In this method, a healthy plant becomes a mother and is left in a permanent stage of vegetation through controlled hours of light. Periodically, a young branch is removed from the mother, treated with a rooting hormone, and planted. The cutting, genetically identical to the mother, becomes a new plant's stem and is allowed to grow and ultimately flower. Through this process, growers can keep their best specimens in perpetuity as mothers and continue popular strains for generations. Growing from a clone is a much faster process than growing from seed and has much more predictable results. As an added bonus, as long as the mother plant was truly a female, clones are guaranteed to also be female.

The Changing Shape of the Cannabis Market

With thousands of strains available on the legal market, and new ones appearing on a near constant basis, a cannabis enthusiast could smoke a new strain every day of the year and never run out of options to try. Growers constantly experiment with crossing strains to develop new varieties with interesting flavor profiles, effects, and size and growth duration benefits.

I spoke with Burt Mackeford (not his real name), a grower who has been working in the industry for 15 years, about his experiences. When it comes to strain selection, he explained, "Strain development is based on several factors: the appearance of a strain, its smell and taste, but most of all, what's in demand. We've developed a following for several strains. If people are loving one of our cookie cuts, we'll breed that with something else people love like one of our OG cuts. It's fun because even when picking from strains we know well, their offspring can throw expressions unlike either parent. We do, however, always keep stock of the things that are our favorites. We still hold strains dating back to the '90s."

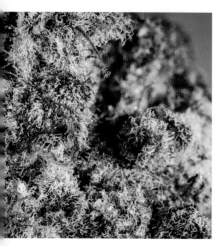
MAC

Where cannabis strain availability was once based on a grower's whim, success now requires as much market research and trend analysis as any other type of commodity. Central to all decisions is the end-user experience and predicting interest based on past successes. According to Mackeford, it's a delicate balance. "We are always researching what is on the horizon. We will pay a lot to obtain things that are in demand before they become popularized. Recently, we obtained a clone of White Truffle, which goes for thousands of dollars per cutting. The hope is to catch on early. We had a clone of Gorilla Glue 4 in 2014 when nobody had any idea what it was. Now it's everywhere."

Some aspects of strain marketing, like naming, are relatively straightforward. Cross Miracle 15 with Alien Cookies, and you get MAC, a title formed by its parents' names. Other aspects are more complex. In a market dominated by existing notions of indica and sativa, each strain must be classified one way or the other regardless of how convoluted the parentage is. Mackeford deals with this regularly in his work. "Determining indica vs. sativa has gotten very difficult with all of the breeding that goes on nowadays. Indicas and sativas will be most pure when coming from a landrace strain. Mostly, we go based on effect, if we are clearheaded, that's seemingly more sativa, while any form of couch lock or sedation goes into the indica category."

Recent massive changes in the technological and legal aspects of the industry have required near constant adaptation for growers. Variability in market pricing, fresh legalization adjusting demand, home growers getting in the game for themselves—it all has had an impact. For growers to keep up and keep the lights on, they need to focus on user experience and create strains that people are destined to love. In many ways, it's a gamble, but for Mackeford, the gamble has been a rewarding one. "My personal use of cannabis has always been intertwined with my work. I use cannabis for back pain, stress, as well as sleep. If I were in pain, anxious, or without rest, I would be less productive. It's also really enjoyable from a recreational standpoint. As someone who loves great food and wine, it is similar in that variety is the spice of life. Cannabis has endless variety."

The User Experience

Cannabis enthusiasts, from the lifelong aficionados to the puff-puff-pass-at-parties crowd, possess a very personal set of preferences when it comes to choosing what and how they imbibe. Method, environment, expectation, and strain are only the beginning for predicting experience outcome.

Smoke It, Eat It, or Dab It?

There are more options than ever to choose from: edibles, tinctures, **wax**, energy drinks, shatter, flower, shake, live resin… You name it; it exists. While many people are excited to try anything and everything with abandon, others prefer to gradually dip a toe into a new method and see what happens. You can always smoke or eat more for an amplified effect.

I gravitate toward smoking or vaping flower. I like to feel awake, and I love to laugh. In my early twenties, I would happily smoke out of a bong, a **hookah**, or even a homemade

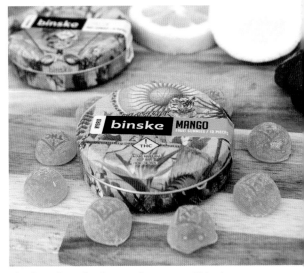

Thanks to broadscale manufacturing, edibles have become much more sophisticated than the brownies your neighbor's boyfriend baked in the '90s.

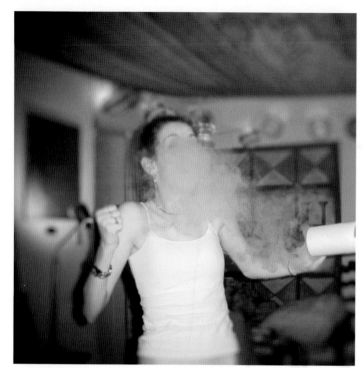

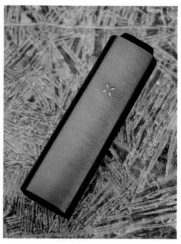

These days, a Pax vaporizer is my preference for a productive high.

College was a time for experimentation with many things, like a four-foot steamroller made out of a mailing tube.

steamroller. I used to love smoking **blunts**, but now they make my eyes too dry, which isn't compatible with computer or camera work. Edibles can sometimes swing too psychedelic and will easily kill a whole day if you're not careful. For me, increased THC levels mean increased paranoia, but CBD-heavy strains don't give quite enough effect. These insights are only a portion of the long list of things I've learned about myself and how I've related to cannabis over the years. Developing personal awareness and preferences is a vital part of the cannabis experience, especially if the goal is to have a productive, creative high.

In their interviews, creatives have shared an extremely wide range of preferences for variety and method of imbibing:

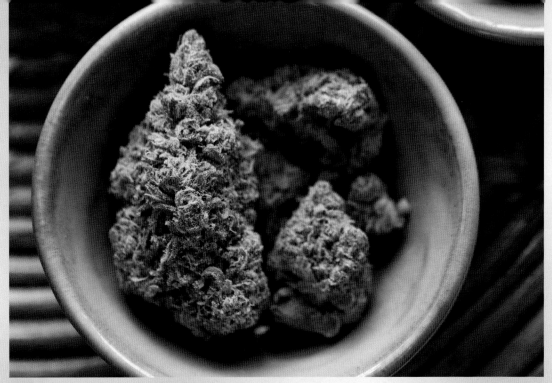

Blue Dream is a popular strain that several interview subjects mentioned by name.

"Smoking flower is my preferred method. I don't like vapes. I hate edibles. I won't get a drawing done if I take edibles. I just want to have a nap. But I like mainly hybrids and indicas. I just get a little more jazzy with sativa. My sober self is already so amped up and always on level 10, so I need that indica to relax [into a creative state]. My favorites are WTF and Sour Diesel."

—JBones,
cartoonist

"It's about how the terpenes work together to affect your body. I could smoke a sativa or an indica before performing, and it wouldn't necessarily make a difference if it was the right blend that I needed."

—Trisha Smith,
musician and performer

"Sativas are definitely more productive for me. If I'm trying to clean my house or something, then definitely sativa. If it's a weekend, and I'm trying to just chill out, then it's more of an indica situation. With art, I feel like it goes both ways because, you know, sometimes I'm trying to make excited art, and then sometimes I'm using it as a way to calm down. So if I'm having an anxious day, I'll have indica so I can relax. When I'm trying to be creative, smoking a joint can get a little out of hand quickly. I get a little too in the mood, and the same with edibles. I want to be alert; I'm not trying to use it to dumb myself down or disconnect. I'm using it to connect. I try to smoke one hit and see how I'm feeling. Maybe have another hit as I go so I can keep that same level of engagement."

—Laurel Williams (not her real name),
visual artist and art teacher

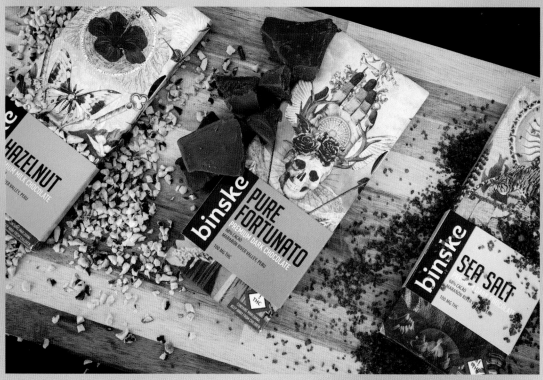

Edibles are easier to transport and consume, but they're not for everybody or every situation.

"Blue Dream was a strain that came around every year at the same time, and I was a big fan of that. I prefer sativa or a hybrid that's sativa dominant because sometimes you do get an indica that just puts you right to bed. It serves its purpose, but it's not what I need it for. If it's a writing session, I like to smoke a joint or even a spliff. I'll throw a little tobacco in there; I'm not above that."

—Uncle Sexy,
   singer-songwriter

"I like joints and being outside when I smoke. It's about connecting outwardly while breathing in and just being alone."

—Nathaniel C. Hunter (not his real name),
   author and activist

"My goal is more for the mental effect than the physical effect. I like how mentally invigorating a sativa is. I like my indicas, too, but that's for a certain time when I'm finished with the millions of things I do throughout the course of the day. As far as strain preference, I like experiencing the variety of flavors and aromas that cannabis has. I love Jack Herrer, and Blue Dream is a good one, but I'm always down to try something new, and I like how diverse it can be."

—Bruno Wu,
   chef

Party of One or The More the Merrier?

For some, pot is an intensely social experience. For others, the best trains of thought can only have one conductor. Often the circumstances and goals for the high dictate which approach is best.

I love to smoke with friends and with my husband. Some of my best witticisms have occurred during group smoke sessions (like my recent revelation that ponies are the corgis of the equestrian world). I also like to start off with friends and then go off on my own for a private creative quest. Other times, I'll happily smoke solo. I enjoy entertaining myself in any state, so why should being high be any different?

Culturally, solo smokers have often faced a stigma that experiencing cannabis alone means that they're somehow more pot-dependent or socially deviant. That couldn't be farther from the truth. Much like it's totally reasonable to sit on your porch and sip a cup of tea or a beer, it's absolutely OK to twist up a joint and enjoy your own company. You don't need other people as an excuse to enjoy pot. It's all a question of how you want to curate your experience and what works best for you.

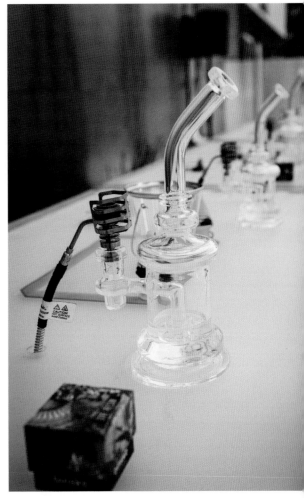

With increasingly more US states legalizing consumption at private events, slick setups like this group-friendly dab bar offer a communal experience outside of smoky living rooms.

"I enjoy smoking with friends and alone too. I love the creative brainstorm energy of a group session. This creative snowball effect happens when you smoke with other people. I also really enjoy my personal process and being able to come up with unique ideas by myself."

—Bruno Wu,
chef

"Smoking isn't very co-creative to me. Even though these things are called 'joints,' which would mean that we somewhat connect…It's never been that way for me. I've always kind of escaped into my own world to an extent that these days I barely ever smoke pot with someone. This might be part of a bigger creation, like dinner and a movie, and a spliff, but normally I do it for myself."

—Juerg "Fed" Federer,
chef, writer, and creativity consultant

"I really love smoking as a group. I have a group of friends with whom I cook and smoke, and it's really nice because we all come from different countries. Every time we get reunited, we cook something different from our countries and then we share this really cultural experience, which is close to our hearts. We smoke, and we eat, and we laugh. It's fantastic."

—Daniela Valdez,
writer and translator

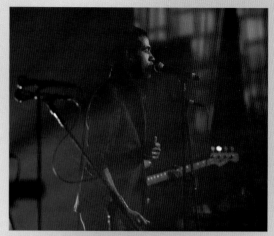

Many of Cassius Wright's favorite lighting looks are inspired by smoke sessions with friends.

"Some of the best lighting design looks that I've ever come up with have come out of hanging out with my friends in smoke-filled rooms with a lava lamp or a cool lampshade casting some strange color in the room. I always use haze if I'm designing with music in mind, so you can really see the shape of the light. A lot of that inspiration comes from smoke sessions. I'm sitting there having a smoke with my friends, thinking to myself, 'Man, this would look really cool in a show one day.' The fact that smoking is a community-driven event has provided me with a lot of those moments that come through in my design work."

—Cassius Wright,
lighting and event designer

CHAPTER 5

CANNABIS AND CREATIVITY: THE INTERVIEWS

In his book, *The Geography of Genius*, author Eric Weiner writes, "Creative breakthroughs almost always require a jolt of some kind, an outside force acting upon our bodies at rest." For many of the creatives presented in the following pages, their cannabis use acts as that jolt in one way or another. Some get high to create; some just prefer being high and happen to be creative. Many connect the creative high to an expansive type of thinking, while others are drawn to the hyperfocused rabbit holes of thought and attention. For many, it's a combination. As you learn about each of these artists, their creative processes, and their relationships with pot, think back to what you now know about creativity, the brain, and the plant that sparked this whole investigation: cannabis.

Note: Refer to the section "Interview Methodologies" (page 34) for information about how I recruited creatives for this project and to see a list of the questions I asked.

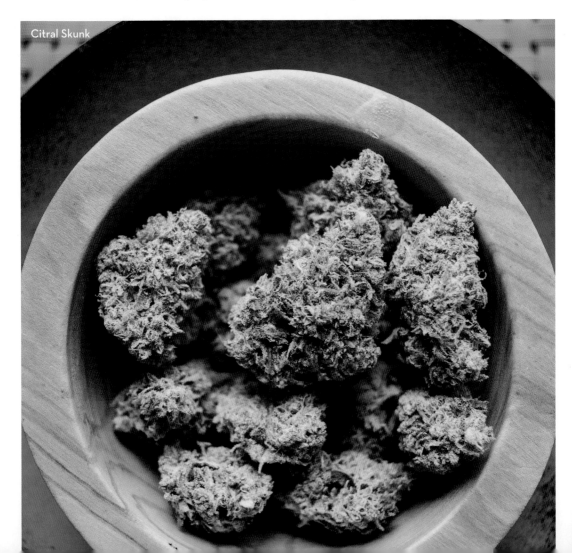

Citral Skunk

Juerg Federer

chef, writer, and
creativity consultant

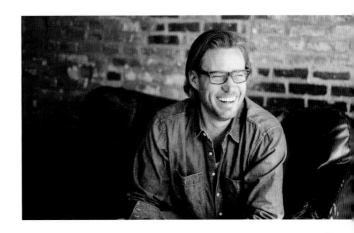

Juerg Federer, who goes by Fed, makes creativity his passion and his business. After a thriving career in the culinary world as a gifted chef—he's the mastermind behind Sex on the Table, a series of 500 sold-out performance dining experiences in New York—he has shifted toward a pursuit of leading others to find their creative stride. Through coaching and mentorship, Fed helps deeply creative people navigate environments that don't always value their outside-the-box approaches.

For Fed, the definition of creation and creativity isn't solely artistic. Life is composed of many moments of creation. He views each decision in our daily existence as an opportunity to create, from choosing to make eye contact with a stranger, creating a connection, to the decision to stay lost in one's own thoughts and create dissociation from the world.

From his home, just outside Zurich, Switzerland, Fed describes some of the challenges many extremely creative individuals face in their lives. Sometimes creativity can be painful, he explains, "Because creativity is an autonomous journey. It's radically individual, whereas the common institutions that regulate our society—like education, talent management in a corporate world, and military—all these social structures are taking all these individuals and forming them into one body. What's painful is when your creativity is so strong that you don't really connect to these systems."

This conflict between inner creativity and the expectation to conform is something Fed has experienced many times in his life, but he's always found a path that aligns with his goals and priorities, like taking the established dining experience and reimagining it as more of an interactive culinary performance.

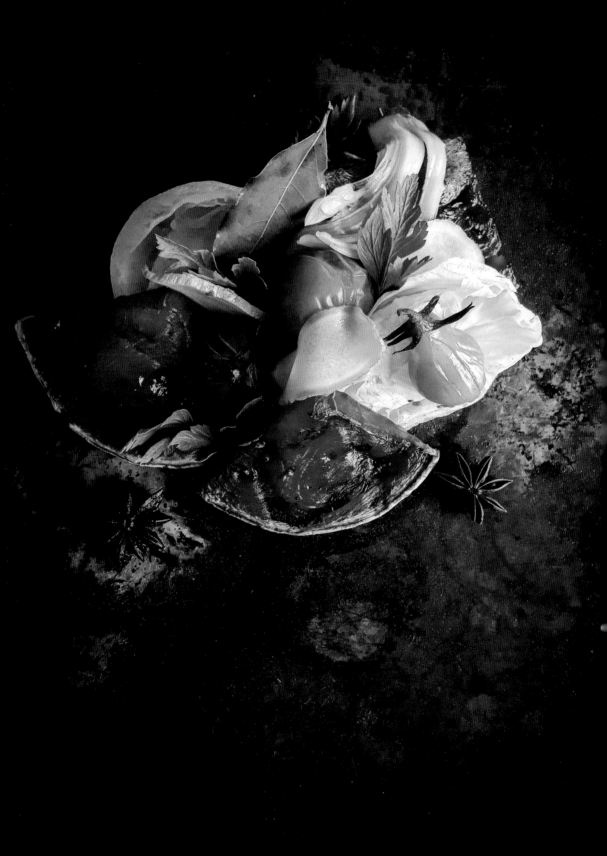

In Fed's personal creative pursuits, he often prefers what he calls "pointless creativity," or creative activities without any particular goal. The simple act of creation helps him feel alive, so he's revisiting his relationship with the cello, he paints horribly (his word) for fun, he cooks at home, and he's writing a novel. Some of these pursuits may end in some sort of identifiable product, while others will simply release some of his creative energy, enriching his existence. In each of these pursuits, the result is less important to him than the experience of getting there.

With that focus on the creative journey, Fed began incorporating cannabis into his pursuits, both personal and professional. Like many cannabis enthusiasts, he had always maintained a strict sense of division between work and play. Cannabis was solely a recreational activity. Then, through food, he came to realize that the inspiration he encountered while high could be valuable for examining flavors, textures, and experiences while cooking and eating.

"I would say food is a very marijuana-friendly business," he tells me. "There's such a rhythm to cooking. It's crazy because first of all, the senses open up when you're smoking pot: your sense of smell, your sense of taste, your sense of texture. These feelings are actually increased, and that really helps in creating a recipe." In his experimentation, Fed found a new drive to go beyond the previously established flavor profiles to create something new and, perhaps, less obvious.

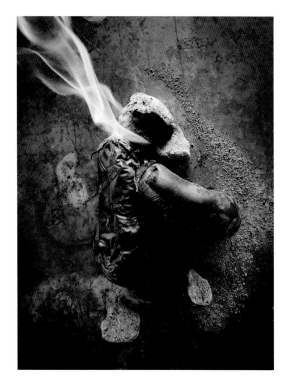

Even the act of serving food at a restaurant is something Fed enjoys with the addition of cannabis. "It has so much to do with a rhythm, a pace that will kind of give you eight arms and legs as you have this 360-degree awareness of what's happening behind you on the stove, what you hear, what you see, what you smell, what you taste...."

Most often, a spliff (his preferred method of consumption) will have the traditionally sought-after result: breaking down mental boundaries and allowing new connections between ideas that have never comingled in his mind before. Other times, smoking will result in the discomfort and paranoia that even the most seasoned cannabis enthusiasts can occasionally experience. With that duality of experience—the elevated and the paranoid—he believes novel creation is more likely to occur.

He explains that, even in its unpleasantness, paranoia can be useful because "if there is no discomfort, we're not going to create anything new because everything is perfect the way it is. You increase your range, your window of response, and therefore you can access the feelings that other people are shying away from."

Though Fed appreciates a wide range of highs, cannabis and creativity aren't necessarily an if–then situation. "I would love for pot to be the switch where you turn on creativity," he says, smiling, "but you know sometimes it's the switch where you turn on couch potato and nothing really happens."

Much like creativity is a personal act for Fed, smoking is usually a solo experience as well. An increase in the flow of ideas both requires and produces a more vulnerable state, so he prefers to work through cannabis-fueled concepts on his own before introducing them to others.

"The creative thought in itself feels like a universe to you, and then you're trying to explain it, and words just don't do justice, but I feel like holding space for a concept—*that's* actually where creativity starts. The biggest enemy of creativity is fear, and when I'm sitting in a room with you and I just birthed this universe, I might be afraid of you destroying it for me, so maybe I'm not willing to show it. I don't need the other person's judgement before my seedling has grown some roots."

Creativity, he explains, is a nebulous concept, evolving throughout our lives. But even in its variability, there are a few key elements that he finds are universally required for being creative: wisdom born of experience, self-motivation to create something new, the courage to fail, individuality outside of institutionalized thinking, and an ideal environment, curated for nourishing the creator while they engage in the vulnerable state of creation.

CANNABIS FOR CREATIVES

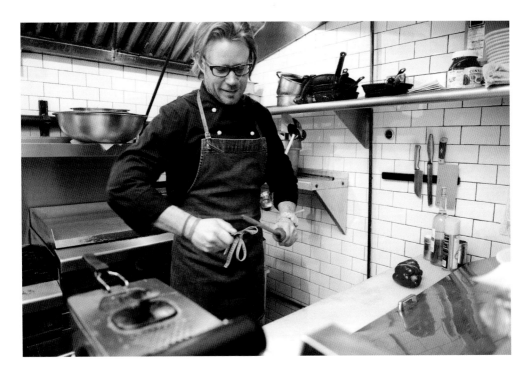

Speaking with Fed about creativity and cannabis is like having access to a contemporary philosopher. His personal reflections on the creative journey, in all its stages, are part of why he is such an effective resource for his clients. "A lot of people who come through my practice are aware that there was a time in their life when they were creative," but the institutions in society, he explains, can break down the natural creative impulse. The goal is to find your way back to the creativity you once knew.

Regardless of cannabis use, environment, or variety of creative pursuit, one thing remains universally true for Fed and all his clients: "The only thing that you never know is when is mother creativity going to access me? You've got to get ready for her."

Ray Benson

musician,
songwriter, and
front man

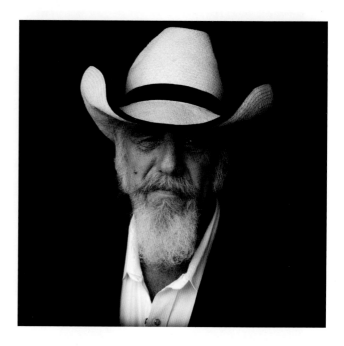

Of all the creatives I had
the pleasure of interviewing
about their relationship
with cannabis, Ray Benson
is perhaps the most high-profile. As the front man (lead vocals and guitar) and founding
member of the popular Western swing band Asleep at the Wheel, Benson's iconic, deep,
yet silky smooth voice has entranced listeners for more than 50 years. Through over 25
studio and live albums, 10 Grammy awards, and thousands of live performances, Benson has
proven that he has no shortage of inspiration and a distinct love of his craft.

JW: I've read some interviews with you over the years, and you've been pretty outspoken about
your appreciation for cannabis, so I thought you might have some good insights to share.

RAY BENSON: I've been smoking pot for 54 years. And have seen the growth of the
information about pot, which is, I think, the one thing that we really desire. I wish they
would let the scientists study it, because when I started [using] pot in early 1967, it was all
Mexican pot or Middle Eastern hashish, and as we learned over the years, they're very
different drugs. They all have different kinds of effects on you. Some pot makes you jumpy,
some pot makes you sleepy, some pot makes you contemplative.... I think the first thing
about creativity is identifying the compounds and what they do to you. And everybody's
different. I tend to like sativa; it gives me an up. Indica makes me sleepy.

One of the areas that the pot helps is that it isolates you. You become very focused. I am,
as my sister would say, a poster child for ADD/ADHD, and pot enables my brain to just slow

down and concentrate on the creative process. The creative process goes on 24 hours a day with folks like me, but when you're jumping, jumping, jumping, which is what ADD is, I've only got 15 minutes of concentration power. People tell me pot's really good for doing housework because you can focus so intently on what you're doing. On the other side of the coin, it can make you very gregarious and very social. It makes things very funny.

I'm a chronic pot user, so it's a different effect. For me, it's a daily medication. I take blood pressure medication and pot. If you are not a chronic pot smoker, when you first smoke, your heart rate goes up. Everything becomes electric. Your senses are heightened; that's what pot does. But if you're a chronic pot user, it's totally different.

JW: Do you remember when you made the connection between cannabis and creativity, where you realized that it might help synthesize thought and put you in a creative mode?

RB: With playing and improvising, whether you're a jazz musician, a bluegrass musician, a blues musician, or a rock musician, when you improvise on your instrument, that's where pot is really helpful because it lets you go places you would never go before. *Or* it traps you in cliché. So, it's not the key to everything, but those are the two things that happen to me when I'm improvising…. It's not the same every time. You start off with some of the same elements and then go. And that's where the best effects of pot happen. Also, in a performance situation, I'm on stage in front of a thousand people. Sometimes I'll go right to what I know because I don't wanna get trapped, but for the most part, absolutely, getting high and improvising is where it's at.

I think sometimes it makes things funny. When you first smoke pot, most people laugh their asses off. Musical humor is something that is inherent in improvisation, so it can certainly enhance that aspect of your improvisation because, "Hey, if I do this, it's musically funny."

JW: Do you think it helps the improvisation if other members of the group are also in that same state of mind?

RB: It's just different, for sure. In my band, the pot smokers interact in a little different way than we do with the non-pot smokers. It's not a positive or a negative. It's just different.

JW: What is your process in terms of writing? Do you have any kind of rituals that you're doing where you plan to write and you smoke first, or do you smoke throughout the day, and it just comes when it comes?

RB: Writing is just the muse, so shoot, a lot of times it's when I'm driving the car. Nine times out of ten, that's where things pop into your head. I sit on this couch, and I have hundreds of notebooks and pads of paper—mountains of them! And I jot things down. Any writer, whether they write novels or they're comedians, anybody, you write ideas down and then you go to work. The inspiration to me is the hardest part, and, as we like to say, the rest is homework.

For instance, we've gotta record next week. I'm sitting on the porch, and all of a sudden there it was. I'm playing a guitar and there it is; I've got a song. I turn on my iPhone or iPad and jot that down. Was it a good idea? Was it stupid? Paul McCartney has the greatest story about him being in a bed and he wakes up. He's got an idea for a song; luckily he has a cassette player.... Boom, and he sings "da-da-da, scrambled eggs, all I want is some scrambled eggs." And that was [the song] "Yesterday," but the inspiration was scrambled eggs. And that's the thing. Every songwriter will tell you they grab the song from the air.

JW: What about when you're performing? Do you smoke before you go on stage?

RB: Yeah. We always have. Me and one of the band members, that's something that we do and feel good about it. It doesn't affect my voice in a negative way, but for some people it's terrible. Some people can't remember what they're doing. If I go into a studio and I'm performing there, I probably smoke less. If we do a show with a symphony where everything is set, you cannot deviate from what's on the page. Then I tend to stay straight or maybe just take a slight hit to, as we say, take the edge off.

In terms of the creativity of what I do on stage, I am the front man. I don't tell jokes, but I'll say funny things, I introduce every song and sometimes have a little banter with the audience. And for that, of course, getting high makes that happen because there's no script. It's about improvising and going places that maybe you wouldn't go if you weren't high.

I was having dinner with Fab Five Freddy. We were comparing experiences of an inner city, hip-hop, Black musician with a baby boomer, country western, hippy musician, and it was very enlightening as to the similarities. People would assume there was nothing in common between these two people, but marijuana, I think, brought the same experiences. And we're very creative people.... I've always said it's a tribal kind of thing, it's a sacrament that's shared by people and creates a tribal communal experience.

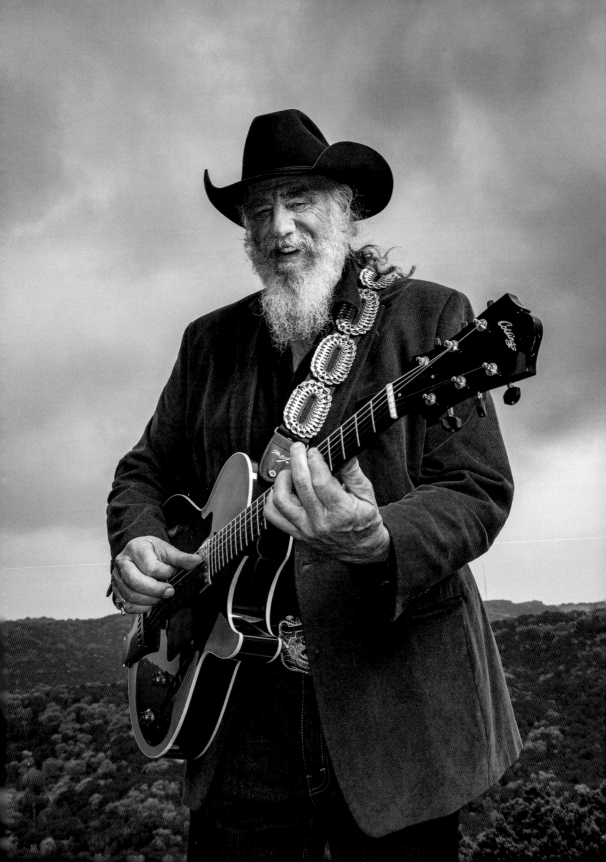

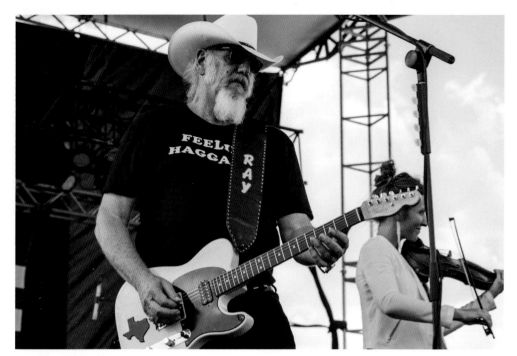

Photo by Nathan Edge.

JW: Do you believe that it's actually making you more creative?

RB: No.

JW: So it's just pulling out what's already there?

RB: Exactly. I could do the same without marijuana. I might not enjoy it, and I'm gonna be different, but different and better aren't the same.

JW: When you smoke, are you smoking joints, or do you use a pipe?

RB: I'm a joint smoker. I tried vaping, I tried. Years and years ago, we knew a guy who had these vape pens, and he made the juice, and it was really good. We were going to Europe, and it was great. I would smoke it on the airplane because you didn't exhale smoke.... And they weren't hip to it either, and we would go through customs and the dogs wouldn't identify it as pot. So it really made our trip very nice through parts of Europe where we couldn't get pot, but it was different. It changes the chemical nature of the marijuana as far as I'm concerned. I'm a joint smoker. I've always liked it, and I know the paper might not be great, but I'm doing pretty good.

JW: Do you like rolling your own joints?

RB: Oh yeah. I make filters and do the whole thing. I started the band in West Virginia, where everybody rolled their own cigarettes. There was an old guy and he had one arm, but he would roll it with one hand. It wasn't good-looking, but it worked. One of the folks in my band was 27 when she joined the band, and she couldn't roll joints. And I said, "You have to learn. It's kind of like driving a stick shift. Sorry kids. There is such a thing." I grow pot myself, I have plants just 'cause I like to do it. And sometimes they're really good. Sometimes they're not.

JW: There's something really meditative about growing and experiencing the whole process. It's a really cool plant.

RB: It's a very amazing plant. I just pulled up three males yesterday, and it's too bad 'cause the males are always big, beautiful, plants. I've grown seeded pot, too, but it's just a pain in the neck. It's just different. But when I was coming up, being here in Austin, it was such a cool thing because it was guys my age in the pot business. It wasn't cartels; it was people. Being a musician, you got to know the dealers. Back in the day, I got Panama Red, got some of the legendary strains that really, really were amazing.

In 1976, there was a guy who came to a show of ours in Lake Tahoe and brought us skunk weed. Literally, it smelled like a skunk. It was purple and green, and he had gotten the seeds and grew it on federal land. It was amazing the way he did it, but it was the first true indica that I ever had. And it literally, it just stunk like a skunk. One of our piano players lived with his mom, and he came back home, and she said, "Tiiiiiim, the dogs must of drug another skunk under the house!" so he had to go take it and bury it outside. It really did stink.

I remember in 1967 going over to a guy's house, a friend of mine, and they had five kinds of hashish: red Lebanese hash, black Afghani hash, this green kief from Morocco, and then this white stuff, and something else—I don't even remember where it was from—it was whitish tan. Our friends would bring back these big bricks with an Arabic stamp on them from Afghanistan. They've been doing this for thousands of years. This is something that is part of their culture. When Vietnam was happening, Thai Stick was some of the best pot. Guys would tell me, "Oh yeah, we used to get what they called OJs from mama-san," and they were opium and marijuana cigarettes. So it's been going on all over the world for years. Obviously, artists use it for inspiration, musicians use it for inspiration…poets, obviously.

JW: What strains do you prefer? Are you selective about it?

RB: Do you mean the names they give it? Give me a break. The names just crack me up.

JW: It's marketing!

RB: I do have a friend, and she breaks it down into indica, sativa, and hybrid. I keep my indica for at night when I'm gonna go to bed. If I play golf, or music, I usually want sativa, but I usually will smoke any joint handed to me and see what happens. And the other thing, the combination that enables you to do that is caffeine. Caffeine and pot are certainly very compatible.

People ask me, "Why pot?" And the answer is because pot enhances your senses. Period. It makes eating more fun, and it's the same thing with music. It really makes playing so much fun. I'm gonna have fun. And if I'm having fun, the audience is gonna have fun.

JW: Is there a single song that you can point to where writing it was an absolute cannabis-fueled experience?

RB: Most of 'em! I mean the good ones. Like I say, the inspiration part is the hard part, and the rest is just homework. I was sitting on the porch and the sun was going down, and I wrote what I think is one of the best songs I ever wrote, and it just flowed out of me. I was stoned, and it was beautiful, and the song just made it. Absolutely. The whole deal is, I pick up a guitar or a pen, or both, or neither, and it starts. That's the creative part. That's total inspiration. And yeah, I like to get high, and I just let it go. And as TJ McFarland, my old friend, said, "If you write a thousand songs, they can't all suck." That's the truth.

Daniela Valdez

writer and translator

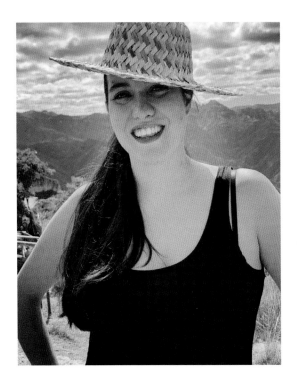

Daniela Valdez is a resolutely independent woman who believes in living well, appreciating the little things, and slowing down to enjoy every moment. Her drive and attention to detail integrate well with her career as a writer, translator, and owner of a small publishing house, Tinta Roja Editoras, in her native Mexico City. About a year ago, Valdez's goal for a slower, more fulfilling life carried her to Spain, where she lives near the beach and spends much of her time outdoors.

Translating and writing, while related in some respects, each involve a unique collection of creative skills. Translating requires a deep understanding of an author's intent and direction, while also capturing not just the literal meaning of the words on the page, but the literary movement, flow, and style. To translate is to interpret without imparting one's own values or biases. It's a pursuit that also requires an absolute mastery of the nuances of each language involved.

At first, translating offered Valdez a way of inhabiting a world of words without needing to expose her own thoughts or literary voice. Translating, like reading, provides an education in written word, plot, structure, and style, all concepts that can help a writer's development immensely. For a budding writer, translating offers a soft transition into creating one's own body of work. "Some people say translators are frustrated writers," she explains. "I didn't

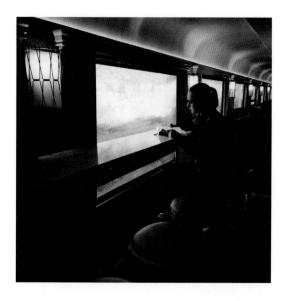

really think so, but I now realize that I was afraid of writing my own work until a few years ago."

Writing original work exposes a greater sense of vulnerability than translating someone else's words. The ideas that writers birth are often entirely their own, and sometimes that can come with conflict and discomfort. For Valdez, the notion of finding her own voice means more than just putting ideas on the page. Her ambition as a writer is deeply connected to her life as an empowered feminist in a culture where women's voices are often given less priority. As her opinions on female equality, environmentalism, and politics grew, she felt more motivated to write. "I think you need to share with the world whatever you have to say, especially as a Latin woman because we live in this macho culture where our voices have always been shut up. Now we have this really vibrant movement which helps us stand up for our rights and talk about our experiences."

Growing more confident with broadcasting her voice and beliefs, Valdez began experimenting with sharing her writing through one of the most direct channels available to her: social media. "As women, we are always told to seek approval. I don't want to do that anymore, so I post whatever the hell I want on Instagram and do my thing."

For her most recent writing projects, she's released single sentences, paragraphs, or movements of a story per day on Instagram. Inspired by the serialized literary format often used by authors of the 19th and early 20th century like Charles Dickens, Fyodor Dostoevsky, and Victor Hugo, Valdez appreciates the idea of engaging her audience with a piece of writing that requires them to slow down a bit. "We are used to what's immediate," she tells me. "We don't have patience. We don't know how to wait for a project to develop or how to wait for the next chapter, so I'm trying to explore that."

Valdez also values cannabis as a means of slowing down and savoring the experiences in her life. Never one to cut corners, she prefers the meditative act of rolling joints over something as simple as using a pipe. "I hate pipes," she says laughing. "Pipes are for lazy people. I think there's something really beautiful about making your own joint. I put some flowers in my joints—lavender or whatever I have growing on my balcony or in my garden. It's really relaxing to make your own joint. It's part of the whole ritual of smoking. If you use a pipe, you lose that magic."

Though she doesn't smoke all the time, Valdez appreciates the way being high allows her to write with more confidence and truth. Smoking silences the inner critic that represents the biggest barrier to her creativity. "I think we all have this ultra-critical voice telling us 'you're not strong enough to do this' or 'you have nothing interesting to say.' Whenever I smoke cannabis, I can shut that voice up and start writing. It's a really nice way to have some empowerment to do the things I love."

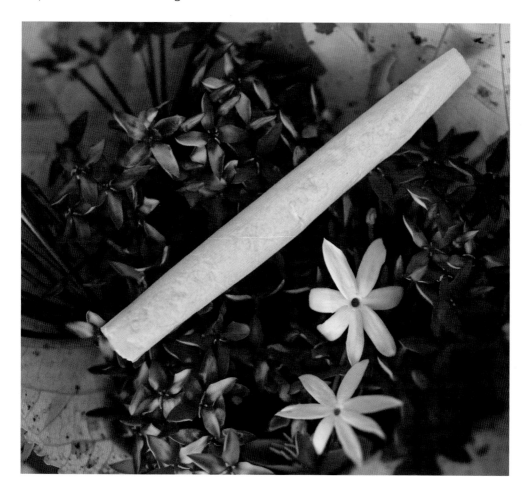

All We Have Is Now—
Short Story/Playlist by Daniela Valdez

Following is an excerpt from a short story Valdez wrote while in a cannabis-fueled creative state. In its original form, she printed the story in a serial format over the course of 33 posts on her Instagram feed.

It was a perfect day for acid. They took the train and went to the beach, holding hands. He loved those days when you really have nothing much to do other than watching the sun rise and set. That is what life should be about: just being.

Just being is bewildering.

Before arriving at the beach, they cut the paper in half and put it on their tongues.

• • •

The place. A beautiful beach in Catalunya. Endless waves, endless clouds. Open space.

There's light beneath your eyes. New overtones in view. Endless form, endless time.

She couldn't really tell apart the songs from her thoughts. The music was messing with her train of thinking. All the textures, all the colors. The blues and whites and pinks and oranges and yellows fading away, melting the sky with the sea. Philip Glass is in the background, "Living Waters." Hi there, Truman. Maybe someone is finally opening that door. Can we stop pretending now?

• • •

The music. Beach House. Foxygen. Deerhunter. Every single bit of psychedelia she could find on the back of her brain. And his favorites on Spotify: Kruaghbin. King Gizzard. Sigur Ros. Hercules & Love Affair. Of Montreal. Alt-J. The playlist named after one of the songs in it: "All We Have Is Now." They had been working on it for weeks. Perfect songs to take acid on the beach.

She had been thinking about it a lot: All we have is now. The present moment. She kept it in mind. He tried to, but could not. She even got it tattooed next to her heart a few months after.

You and me were never meant to be part of the future.

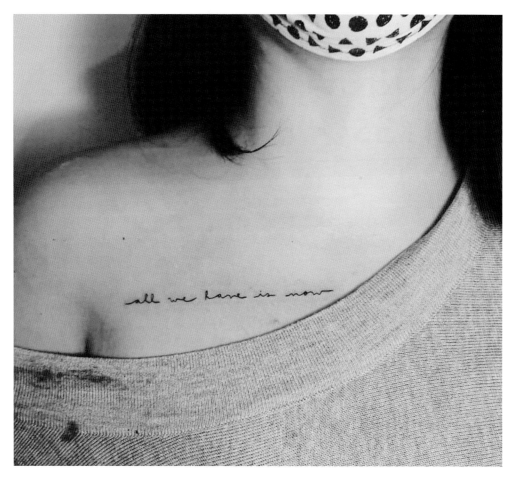

Yet my hands are shaking, I feel my body reeling.

So there they were, watching the wonders of nature.
The wonders of feeling the air when it touched her body,
just staring at the sea.

• • •

The acid was whispering some lyrics to him. But also colors,
and textures. The music was speaking lyrics in colors.

Whatever colors you have in your mind. I'll show them to
you, and you'll see them shine.

To read the full story, scan here.

To listen to the accompanying
playlist, scan here.

Michael Marras

sculpture artist

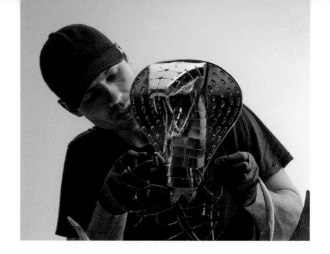

In both his journey with creativity and his experiences with cannabis, sculpture artist Michael Marras learned early that conventional constructs in education and life didn't quite fit the path he was meant for. He remembers a brief spark of early fulfillment in grade school when his teacher let the class turn their sterile classroom into a rainforest. It was magical: a place where he wanted to spend time and enjoyed learning. Other teachers complained, fire code was cited, and the classroom rainforest was quickly dismantled. After that, the classroom felt even more stark for Marras because he had seen the possibility of what it could have been.

Like many children who grow up to be artists, Marras felt his best while finding ways to apply his imagination and creative skills, but beyond elementary school, artistic opportunities became fewer and farther between. He found school to be an uninviting place where creativity was allowed to languish. Add to that a diagnosis of ADD and a hefty prescription of Adderall to help him focus, and he felt distant, unchallenged, and disinterested in what school had to offer.

Ironically, Marras first found pot through his school's D.A.R.E. program. He and his friends had always believed the stereotypes that drug dealers were unapproachable, threatening, or dangerous. In the D.A.R.E. program, Marras was warned that drug dealers would try to be his friend to sell him drugs, which immediately made dealers seem less scary and far more approachable. He and his friends visited what was commonly known to be a neighborhood drug house, bought some pot, and started experimenting.

In high school, smoking pot offered a way for Marras to focus and get through his day at school without any of the problematic side effects of the ADD meds. He was convinced.

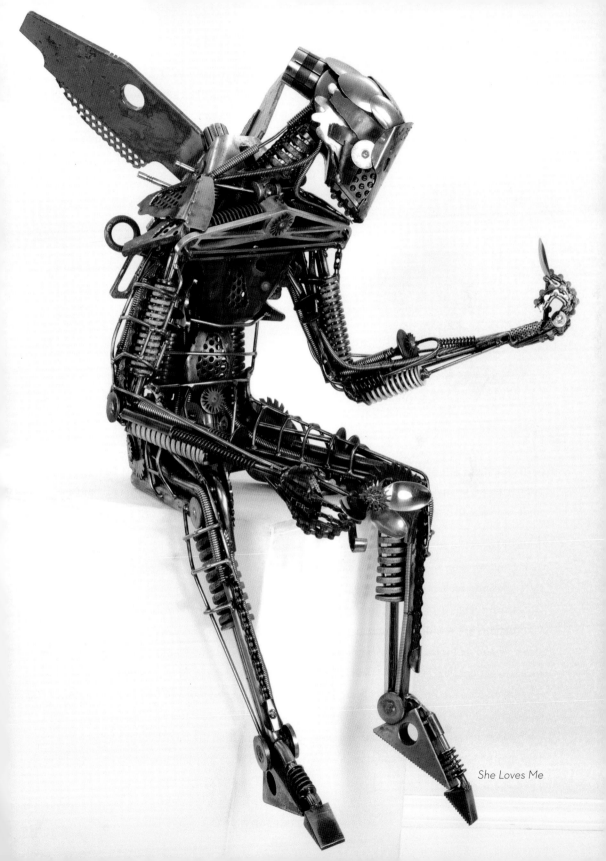

She Loves Me

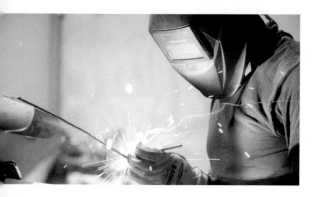

"I realized that for me it was better than the pills. I didn't like how they made me feel. If I had the right cannabis, I could pay attention for as long as I wanted, but I would still want to eat food and I could sleep at night." Marras laments that doctors jumped to pharmaceuticals to manage his ADD and wishes that medical cannabis had been an option. He explains, "I think about what would it have been like if there was a doctor who had said 'Oh, if we give you this strain and you have this much at this time, and this much at that time,' and it was regulated and talked about, how much of a difference that could have made for me. It could have made a big difference for my teachers, too, because I wasn't great to teach. I was just extremely unhappy."

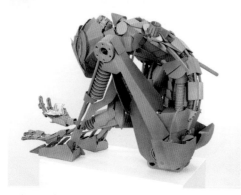

Rebirth of Goji

What his education lacked in creative outlets, he made up for in his free time. His parents supported his artistic impulses with a steady stream of art supplies, trips to museums, and an understanding that he preferred imagining characters and worlds over algebra homework.

Today, Marras is a successful and driven artist who brings his creative imaginings into reality. Living and working in Los Angeles, he spends his time inventing and fabricating highly detailed, large-scale metal sculptures. He calls his body of work "Mythrobotic." Drawing from Greek mythological influences (he's of Greek descent) and a futuristic, robotic aesthetic, his creations are wonderfully rich in gesture and emotion, and his process is incredibly strategic and methodical. While he does source materials for some pieces at junkyards, recent creations, like his piece "Tiger Shark," involve an extreme level of planning. To save fabrication time on the back end, Marras planned and designed much of that project on the computer, ultimately ordering 146 pieces of cut aluminum and steel from a CNC vendor. Each piece arrived, cut perfectly to his specifications, and then the painstaking, 26-day assembly process began. Not bad for a kid who had problems focusing in school.

In Marras's professional career, cannabis has continued to provide a helpful means of concentration. When he gets tired or feels burned out, a few hits on a bowl will put him back in the zone, and he can happily continue to work for a few more hours. "It definitely helps me physically and mentally push on and just get into this other state, this other level. The first eight hours of working, it's very meditative; then I go into this other level where I'm not even thinking about the work. Everything is kind of blank, and I'm moving from one step to the next."

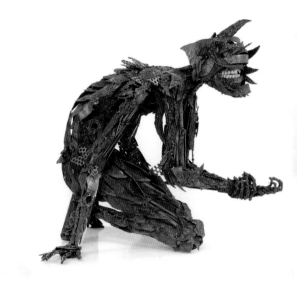

Cryza; The Pitts of Woodruff

In his experience, cannabis is more appropriate for some applications than others. When he's writing stories for the characters he creates, pot makes it harder to focus. He finds that he forgets all his training in writing techniques, so he's rarely happy with what he's written while stoned. But when it comes to imagining storylines, characters, and worlds, smoking helps

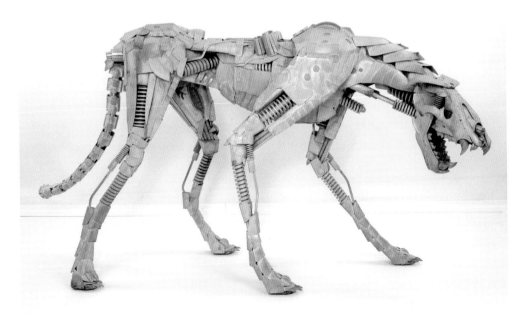

Wolfboy; The Search for Goji

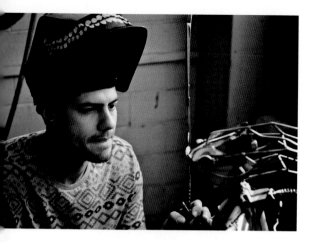

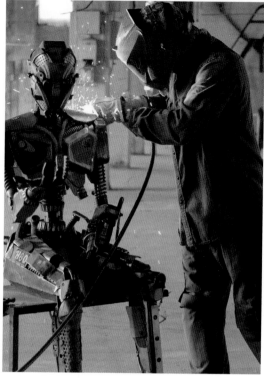

him access his creative muse. Pot doesn't create his ideas, but it helps him find ways to support and develop his ideas further.

Occasional month-long breaks from smoking provide important time for reflection and clarity. He credits his level of introspection and personal accountability with taking the time to think about his life and his work from a position of clear-headedness. He doesn't want to get to a point where pot is his all-day, everyday state of mind. It's a tool with a specific purpose. He explains, "I personally recommend that people take long breaks, especially if they've been smoking forever. I've found that quitting brings all the stuff back that I never processed when I was high. Stuff I never thought through. Once I'm in a good place with those things mentally and I've worked through them, then I can come back to cannabis. I'm using it in a way where it's not about blocking emotions. Every time I take a break, I think it creates even more potential for what pot can be in my creative process."

In his work, Michael Marras likens pot to Dumbo's feather. He can fly without it, but it's nice to have as a reminder of creative possibility. "I have this," he tells me, holding up his own imaginary feather. "It's gotten me places, but it's not necessary one way or another. I know exactly what it will do, so I can choose to use it or not, but now I'm in more control of the process, knowing how it's going to work to my benefit."

CANNABIS FOR CREATIVES

Carlos Mandelaveitia

art director

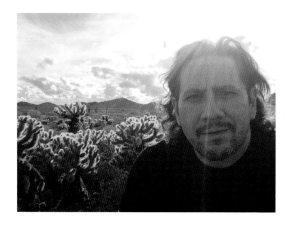

With an education in art and an inner directive to help artists achieve their goals and find their voices, Carlos Mandelaveitia is the cofounder and senior creative director at Divi Media in Cave Creek, Arizona. He is a driving force behind the scenes, engaging with artists, photographers, galleries, and museums to provide branding, sophisticated website development, digital imaging, and custom, large-format print production for gallery and museum exhibitions. Endlessly approachable, Carlos gave off an energy of instant warmth and camaraderie. Talking about art is what he loves to do, and cannabis only enriches the process.

JW: Can you give me some background on your artistic journey: what it is you do, how you arrived there, how you define yourself as an artist?

CARLOS MANDELAVEITIA: I work as an art director. I work with artists, to help bring their visions to life. I do a lot of projects for the museums and galleries out here. I do all the large-format printing and digital work. I don't do mass production type stuff; I work with limited artists that want perfection. And I'm somewhat anal-retentive in that aspect.

I used to consider myself an artist, I used to paint and draw, do pen and ink, you name it, but many years ago, I had an apartment fire and it wiped out everything that I've ever created. Since then, I've pretty much been commercial. I don't consider myself an artist, even though my entire life revolves around artists. I take photographs, but usually it's when I have another photographer who says, "Hey, you're coming with me."

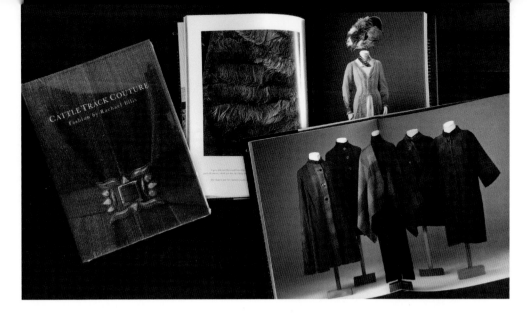

JW: Do you feel a creative impulse for the work that you're doing with other artists? Is it creatively fulfilling for you?

CM: It is! I enjoy it. I've always enjoyed being on the back end of things; I've never been one for the limelight. I'm one of these people who will work on museum shows or gallery shows, and everybody kinda knows me, and wants to talk, but after about 10 minutes, I'm ready to hightail it. I'm definitely an introvert. My goal in life is to be a happy hippy hermit.

JW: What do you think the relationship is between cannabis and creativity? Do you think they're connected?

CM: I think it can help, for sure. There's definitely a balance. The vast majority of the artists I work with partake in something, whether it's mushrooms or weed or something else. From my experience, smoking for the last 30 years, it definitely helps relax the mind. For instance, in the commercial work that I do, you're being pushed against deadlines. Creativity doesn't necessarily just turn on and off, so when things aren't flowing, go enjoy a little break, let your mind wander. That's where I find the most benefit. Instead of having a linear thought pattern, pot opens up my relationships to how things *can* be. That's where creativity enters.

I also see how for a lot of artists it can be a detriment because they get lost in just being high for a while, and nothing gets done. They may be *creative*, but nothing gets *created*. And I've been there, especially in the evenings when you're trying to wind down, you partake a little bit more than you normally would. Then your mind is just going. But unless I'm writing things down, that entire creative mindset kinda gets lost.

JW: When did cannabis come into your life?

CM: I was probably 14. I'm 50 now. So a while ago.... But back then, it wasn't the same. Back then, you could smoke, and you get that little happy high and cough a lot, and you were good. Now you pick up some stuff, you take a couple of puffs and you're sitting for an hour. It's nice, but then you have to take the creative mind flow and make it a reality—bring it into your working world and actually make it flow.

JW: Is that something that's more difficult with the increased potency?

CM: It depends on the strain. Some sativas that should lead to a flow, don't. And some indicas that should put you down actually work the opposite for me and just light up my brain. But once you find the right strain, smoking is very useful, especially if you're interacting with someone and you're trying to hash out ideas. It allows me to verbalize a few more things that I would normally just keep to myself. It reduces that inhibition a little bit, and you're a little bit more blunt about things. Which makes things move through a lot easier.

JW: Do you remember when you made that transition from smoking "weed is fun" to "smoking weed can be a productive state that fuels what you're trying to do"?

CM: When I started smoking weed, it was for fun. Even in art school, it was for fun, but we were all in the same place, and we were all very highly motivated, so while we were having this fun, we were being creative, and it just kind of naturally progressed in that direction.

JW: You've touched a couple of times on the communal experience of collaborating creatively. Do you think it helps if everyone's on the same page?

CM: I've been lucky, being in the art world, most of my clients partake. I don't think I have any clients, even corporate clients, that don't know I'm a pothead. But all the jobs get done above and beyond what they want, so they don't care. Me being stoned works for them.

I definitely see it as a benefit when everybody is partaking or at least in a relaxed state. We had a studio downtown, and we had a nice little sitting area outside with trees. My clients would come over with weed, and we would sit outside and smoke and chat for an hour before we started the project. That was just normal practice.

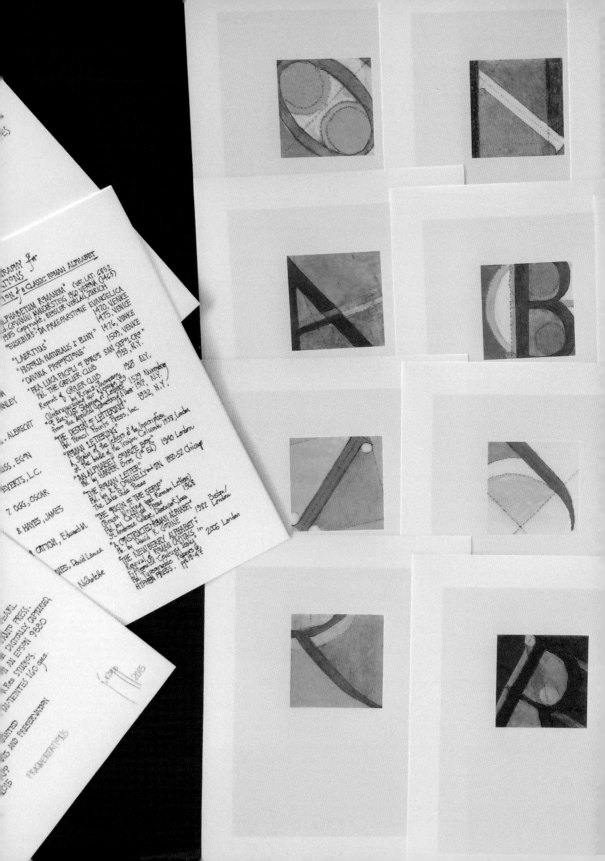

...RAPHY for
...TIONS"

...ION of a CLASSIC ROMAN ALPHABET

"ALPHABETUM ROMANUM" (VAT.LAT. 6852)
...o GIOVANNI MARDERSTEIG, 1G2 VERONA (1463)
1985 Copyright, BESSLER VERLAG, ZURICH

"EUSEBIUS"·DA PRAEPARSTIONE EVANGELICA
                                    1470 VENICE
                                    1475, VENICE

"LAERTIUS"   1476, VENICE
"HISTORIA NATURALIS of PLINY"   1509, VENICE
...INLEY
"DIVINA PROPRITIONE"   SAN SEPOLCRO
                                    1933, N.Y.
...,ALBRECHT "FRA LUCA PACIPLI of BORGOS
        Pbl. THE GROLIER CLUB   1933 N.Y.
        Reprint of our (MASTROS) 1527 Nuremberg
            by Paul Thompsons of 1917, N.Y.
...SS, EGON (Undergroundsound our (GESTAS)
        "THE LOST SCIENCE of TRUTH" 1932, N.Y.
        from the Ancient Geometry
...EVERTS, L.C. "THE DESIGN of LETTERING"
            Pbl. Pencil Points Press, Inc.
        "ROMAN LETTERING"   1939 London
...Z OGG, OSCAR A Study of the Letters of the Inscription
            at the base of the Trajan Column 1940 London
...8 HAYES, JAMES "AN ALPHABET SOURCE BOOK" (1st ED) 1950·52 Chicago
                Pbl. by HARPER Bros
        "THE ROMAN LETTER"
            Pbl. by R.S. DONNELLYand SN 1950·52 Chicago
                The Lake Side Press
...CATLICH, Edward M. "THE ORIGIN of THE SERIF"
            (Brush Writing and Roman Letters)
                Pbl. THE Catfish Press   1968
                St.Ambrose College Davenport,Iowa

...RIES, David Lance "A CONSTRUCTED ROMAN ALPHABET" 1982 Boston/
                by David R. STONE   London
...Nichalelle "THE NEWBERRY ALPHABET"
            Revival of ROMAN CAPITALS, in 2005 London
            Pbl. Turanoodle Papers (J)
                HYPHEN PRESS, 1979·97

FROMP 2015

JW: That sounds amazing. Do you find that artists are more open to feedback on their work or feel less defensive if they're high?

CM: Absolutely. Because immediately, it's a much more relaxed state. It isn't just the mental state from being high—you're in a friendlier environment. When you're high, you're not really performing, you're just kind of relaxing and being yourself and interacting. Some of those masks come off and make the process easier.

JW: Where does pot fit into your life? Are you somebody who just gets up and smokes, and creativity happens simultaneously with being stoned, or do you smoke when you intend to work?

CM: I wake and bake. Well, I should restate that. I don't bake. I wake and *toke*. On an average day, I'm a toker. Right now, I'm working out of the house. I have a nice home studio. I have a big property that I can just walk around, and it hasn't been 120° yet, so I can enjoy it. When I go out, I'll go toke, but I won't get stoned. Then I get back to work.

I'm always very conscious as to which strain I have, depending on what type of work I'm doing. For instance, if I'm doing website coding, my brain needs to be fairly focused. Not just strain related, but I know I can't just take a few too many hits, because any little thing will mess up the coding. So it's just enough to help with the focus. Other times when I'm doing digital imaging and cleaning up 30 images for a show, I get hyperfocused, which is beneficial. I can be pretty taken by the smoke and produce a very good product. It's always related to what I'm doing. There are days that I don't smoke at all. I don't have to; I just kind of like to. If I don't have any, I don't freak out. There's a weird balance there.

JW: Can you describe what it feels like when you've smoked?

CM: It does help with pain. I was diagnosed with fibro[myalgia], and it definitely helps with the intensity. I also do CBD. When you're in front of a computer looking over, feeling like a giraffe, it helps with all of that tension. It just kind of eases it. But the biggest benefit I see is mental. For me, it's almost like doing a little bit of meditation to help quiet the mind and refocus. Working on a number of projects at once, I always have that distracting voice, "Oh, you gotta get this one," or "You gotta look at that one." You take a toke, and you just refocus on what's in front of you, and that's very beneficial.

JW: Are there other rituals or things you're doing to set yourself up for creative success?

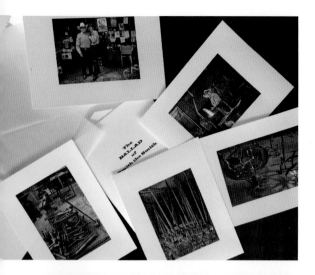

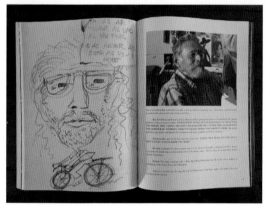

CM: The biggest thing that I do is focusing on taking breathers. In the evening, I will toke and then I will meditate with whatever I want my mindset to be and go to bed. I find that helps a lot upon waking. You're no longer stuck in certain merry-go-rounds of thought. Pot helps with that process. Years ago, I was certified as a clinical hypnotherapist. One of the things that I did is I created a trigger for myself, so when I get stoned, I just initiate the trigger and within a minute I'm in a good state of meditation. I don't have to go through this ritualistic tuning down because the weed has relaxed me enough, so once I engage the trigger, I just go straight into meditation.

JW: That's cool! So what does the trigger look like?

CM: A trigger can be anything, but for me, I use two fingers and I tap my knee in a certain rhythm, and that initiates the overall sensation. It's kind of like you program yourself to go from here straight to there. You know what the center feels like because you've experienced that, so the trigger allows you to get from point A to point D real fast.

JW: How are you imbibing? Do you always smoke?

CM: I've tried everything. Clients give me things. So, I have syringes of concentrates, I have little pieces of wax…. You name it, I've got it. I enjoy the smoke. I enjoy having a joint, but the new stuff is so expensive, you don't want to roll it. The only time I do edibles is when I'm looking to just chill for the day. If I actually have some time off and I just wanna forget about the day or forget about the weekend, then I'll do the edibles, because I find they really do stay in my system.

JW: OK, so what strains in particular do you tend to gravitate toward?

CM: You know, nowadays almost everything is a hybrid. But I'll do a sativa-dominant for the day, and I like an indica-dominant for the evening. As far as a particular strain, probably my favorite is New York Sour Diesel. Most of the OG Kush type stuff is fine, or Gorilla Glue.

JW: Gorilla Glue is a sleeper! Can you stay awake on that?

CM: Oh God, yeah, I love that stuff. See, that's one of the ones that, yeah, it relaxes you, but it actually pops up my mind.

JW: That's one of the things that's been so interesting about these interviews, is seeing just how many different responses people have to the same strains. If I smoke a Gorilla Glue, I'm done. Nothing else is happening that day….It's great that you've found what works for you.

CM: For the most part, I think cannabis is a very beneficial substance. I started doing cannabis to get myself off of the medication that I was prescribed for the fibro. I took it for about a year, and the entire time I was taking it I felt like a zombie. It was not good for me. I decided I can't live that way. So I started dosing a little bit more with cannabis and with CBD, and it controlled the symptoms much better than the medication. I know from my own experience that cannabis can help a lot of individuals dealing with pain. A lot of the pain medications just wipe you out. So there is no creativity, there's nothing. There's a numbness. So between having that numbness from a little pill in a bottle or smoking some weed? I'd much rather smoke weed, have more relief, have a sense of creativity, and not a sense of something controlling me.

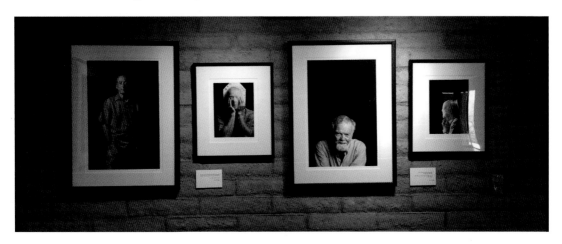

Christopher O'Riley

pianist, arranger, and composer

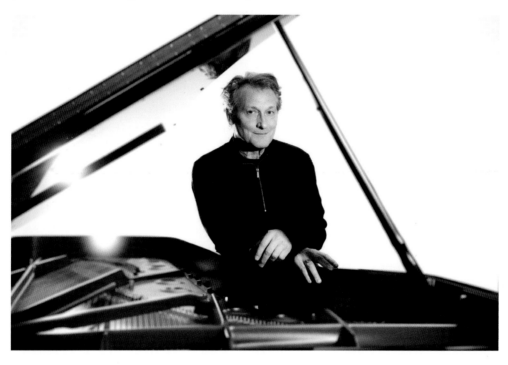

As an artist who makes his living and his art with his hands, Christopher O'Riley, pianist, media personality, and audience-beloved former host of NPR's *From The Top*, carries a conversation with subtle and lyrical hand gestures. Ideas and motions go together as if, in the act of expressing his insights, he's conducting an invisible orchestra of thought.

Best known for his piano arrangements, recordings, and performances of popular music in the contemporary canon—think Radiohead, Nirvana, Elliot Smith, and Nick Drake—O'Riley approaches his transcription work through immersive study and experience. He relates his musical explorations as being "discovery-oriented" rather than "task-oriented." To create one of his piano interpretations, he begins by listening to the original track on repeat. Through an almost obsessive immersion into a song, he's able to draw out the essence of it while simultaneously composing other musical trains of thought that enhance and engage the original. Think of it as a musical conversation. A call and response. Echoes and explorations.

"Usually, it's like picking at a thread. I think the best example is that sort of mandala guitar line that begins "Let Down" by Radiohead. That's part of the texture, and then I add other textures. It's a fractal process. It's focusing but also panning back," he explains, his words punctuated by an almost palpable energy held between his palms.

A single recording of a track is enough for O'Riley to examine in his way, but when multiple recordings exist, that's when he really thrives. "Solo versions, early versions, late versions, things that an artist recorded at home—all of these become ways into the music, but they also become resonances. The more ideas I collect, the more special moments I can explore. I hoard all these beautiful moments, and at a certain point it becomes a matter of chipping away. Like Michelangelo making a sculpture, you reach a point where you're chipping away everything that isn't the piece. It takes a long time to get to that point, but it's a beautiful feeling."

Accessing the right creative energy for his work involves a combination of curated mental states. As a self-proclaimed endorphin junkie, much of the time he spends bathing in a piece of music occurs while on his exercise bike, or his stair machine, which he recently, very literally, wore into the ground. A more contemplative state, achieved through predawn meditation practices and a love for cannabis, also helps him focus his creative energy. "Meditation and cannabis open a portal of possibility. I think the more consistently I meditate, the more consistently I have more forward thinking and new ideas."

As with many artistic prodigies, piano has been a part of Christopher O'Riley's life since the age of four. From childhood classical piano lessons, through self-guided studies of jazz and rock and roll, to formalized classical conservatory training, O'Riley's formative years were spent in pursuit of music. Inspired by the artists of his teens and early twenties, he sought a way to fuse the emotion and familiar melodies of popular music with his "piano musings." His expansion of popular compositions coincided with the expansion of his creative mind through the selective enjoyment of pot. In describing his experiences when high, O'Riley says, "I realized that it was having this sort of focusing while defocusing effect, and that my presence at the piano, physically, mentally, and emotionally was enhanced by spare use of the drug."

For the best creative energy, O'Riley practices moderation. "I've never been more than a one-hitter. If something is so strong that it really incapacitates me, I'm just not interested, but if it makes me happy and doesn't cause me to lose any capacity, then it actually feels to me like a threshold of understanding and awareness."

Though O'Riley never performs or records his music while stoned, he appreciates the way cannabis enhances the process of immersing in a piece and developing his transcriptions. "I'm always interested in the lateral sort of thinking. Something occurs to me, and then I end up down a very splendid rabbit hole, a possibility that I wouldn't achieve if I was very directed and Type A about it. That's the kind of way my mind works naturally, so it's a matter of trying to encourage that openness and being in the moment."

With an encyclopedic knowledge of music from the classical to the contemporary, O'Riley is well aware of the historic relationship between music and altered states of consciousness. In 2018, he performed in Basil Twist's acclaimed New York revival of *Symphonie Fantastique*, a live, aquatic, puppet-based interpretation of Hector Berlioz's 19th-century, five-movement composition.

"*Symphonie Fantastique* was basically written as an opium hallucination. Basil Twist staged it in a huge fish tank with lots of colored lights and pieces of fabric, these sort of ghosts that were going through this aquarium, and it was like a fantasy taking place in front of you, except that there were five puppeteers in wetsuits, splashing away backstage, and I was at a Steinway in front, standing in for the composer."

Through movement, color, light, and O'Riley's nuanced performance on the piano, the production encapsulated Berlioz's opium-fueled, musically depicted story of unrequited love, fantasy, obsession, and murder. Contemporarily, some may tend to think of drug-induced creativity as a more recent phenomenon, but O'Riley explains, "This whole symphonic work, written three years after Beethoven died, is a complete hallucination. So it's been around for a while."

While Berlioz's exploration of opium depicted the darker, more macabre side of altered consciousness, O'Riley prefers the light, energetic, and thoughtful results of Blue Dream and other sativa strains. In his years of cannabis use, he has learned that variety is important for his creative highs, as is the ability to embark on new ways of thinking about and achieving old goals.

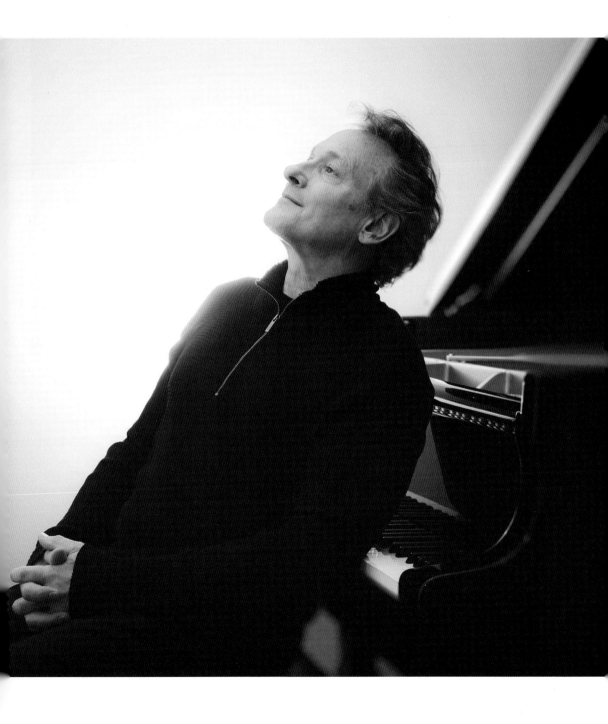

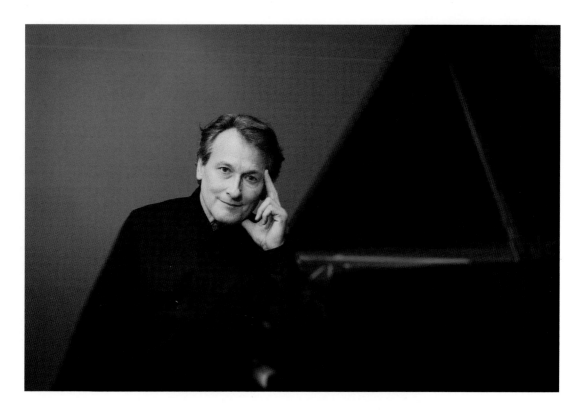

"To a large extent, both meditating and cannabis encourage relinquishing the reins of control. I don't think it's necessary in order to be creative, but it is an enhancement. I've been on a continuous upward trajectory in terms of learning and new ways of preparing for performance. That comes from both ways of living: one very disciplined, very sober, and one slightly more enhanced. I think everyone has to find their own path."

That interest in self-direction and flow of experience has always defined Christopher O'Riley, both in his career and in his creative approach to music. He excels at guided assignments and gigs, but the opportunities to follow his own creative musings always seem to result in something unexpected and compelling, not just for audiences, but for his own personal creative satisfaction.

Garrett Shore

multidisciplinary artist

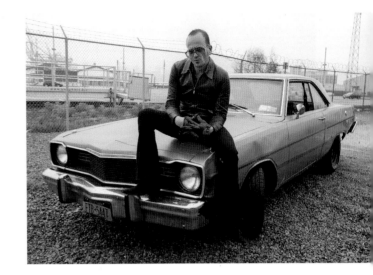

Garrett Shore is a New York City–based artist and professional tour guide. For over 13 years, Shore has engaged and educated NYC visitors with his carefully crafted, detailed, and compelling historical walking tours of the city. He's known for infusing humor, providing unique and fascinating historical context, and keeping an upbeat energy during his tours. Shore's tour guide work actively incorporates the same creative energy and attention to detail that he utilizes in his musical and visual arts pursuits.

JW: Can you start by introducing a bit about who you are and what sort of creative pursuits you explore in your life?

GARRETT SHORE: There's an old expression: jack of all trades, master of none. Well, I am a jack of many artistic pursuits and a master of none. I cannot juggle art in that I can't be writing music at the same time that I'm making a film, or at the same time I'm making collages or photography. I will divert all of my mental energy into one and forgive the crass nature of what I'm about to say, but I think of it in terms of a libidinal force. It's like a horny-ness for achieving a very specific either visual or audio thing. I'll feel satisfied with that, and then I'll ruminate on the pointlessness of things that exist purely as audio experiences or as visual experiences, and I want something that has a very literal meaning, so I'll get really excited about making a film or writing. It's sort of like a season, you know how you've got winter, spring, summer, fall. I've got music, filmmaking, photography, and sometimes collage.

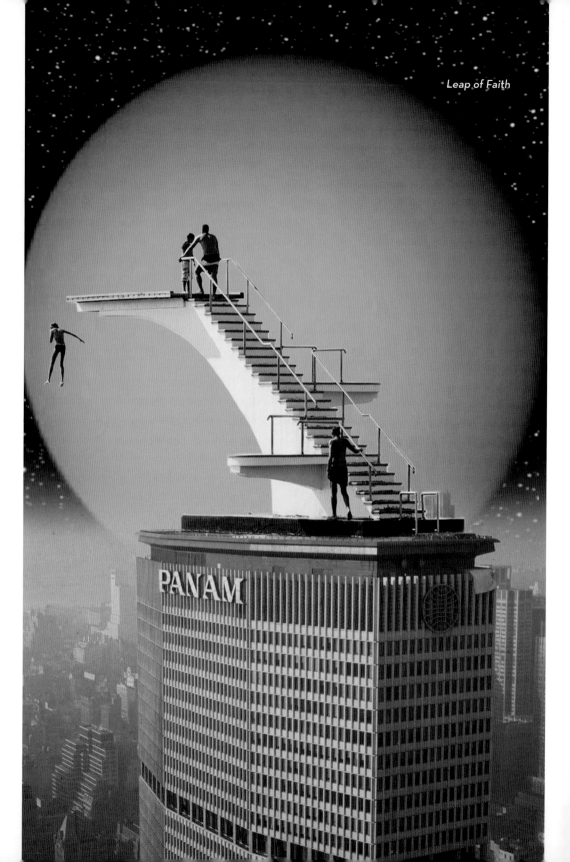

Leap of Faith

JW: What inspires you to work in each of those directions?

GS: Some people are just naturally creative. I'm not. I'm naturally analytical. My natural tendency is to look at things and question them, and I think of creativity along those lines. Mozart didn't think that he was an artist; he thought that he was an instrument and that God was the artist. That's a very sincere claim of belief. I think of it as if there is a well that your creative spirit draws from. You take the bucket, and you stick it in the well. But what brings the water to the well? I'm more extroverted than I am introverted. Most of my inspiration comes from being surrounded. That's why I love being in New York City. There's a human energy that I draw from.

JW: Do you gravitate toward one medium more often? I have always really enjoyed your photography.

GS: There's something meditative about photography. I think the most amazing things about photography are the processes. I love the methodical nature of it. With music, you have to play the right notes, and if you're not playing the right notes, it sucks, but with photography, everything has potential. There's a visual language. I love exploring that, and I love the meditative nature of working in Photoshop. There are so many people that are better than me by such a country mile that I don't get a sense that anything I could ever do would be that interesting or that unique, so it all just seems very futile. When I go on Instagram, and I don't do it frequently 'cause it's a frustrating way to communicate with people, I find there's something demeaning about it. It's like, I don't want you to just scroll, I want you to *look*. But it's also understandable because there's so much content to sift through.

JW: I know what you mean. It almost feels like people dancing in windows in the red-light district in Amsterdam. Trying to catch attention as spectators are walking by, and if you don't attract enough people then you must not be that talented. But passing appreciation on Instagram is never enough to actually indicate the work that goes into it: the intent, the creativity, and the knowledge base that you developed over time.

GS: So many fish in the sea artistically resonate right now that it's impossible to stand out. I feel that our generation is in an art desert, even though we are in this free-for-all of content, and it's because we are more connected than ever, yet we know less and less how to actually communicate with one another in an enriching way. I think most of the best art that's out there right now is made in the pursuit of self-satisfaction and not audience satisfaction.

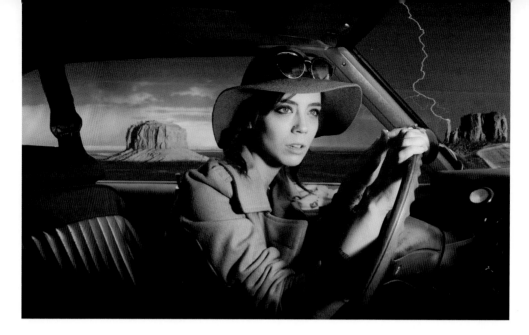

JW: Let's talk a bit about cannabis. I'm curious to see how it fits into your philosophies about art. When did pot come into your life, and what has it been for you over the years?

GS: The first time I smoked was maybe when I was 14 or 15. They say weed is stronger now, but back then my mind was much more receptive to an experience. It felt like it was being pried open like a chestnut. Do you know what I mean? All the infinite possibilities made the idea of being high very alluring 'cause it's this expansive thing. All these years later, I don't smoke weed often, but when I do, I don't smoke it to expand anything; I actually smoke it to withdraw or to narrow my focus. I only smoke indica. I don't like things that make me jittery. Sativa makes me think in cycles. I get propeller-like thoughts that can keep going and going and going. Indicas are much more about relaxation. Also, I do not ever smoke marijuana socially. If I'm out and somebody offers, I never accept because I know that if I smoke in a social setting, as soon as I get high, the first thing I'm gonna think is, "I need to get out of here." It will instantly change the dynamic; it'll bring me directly into introvert mode when I was at the party having a good time, being in extrovert mode.

JW: Has it always been that way?

GS: Yes, I don't think I've ever smoked weed and been more sociable. When somebody else is talking, I won't listen. I'm not as good at being a friend to people, and I'm just more withdrawn.

JW: So what's your ideal use for it?

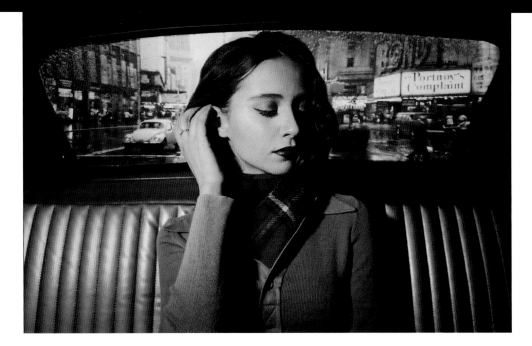

GS: I think the best way to describe my relationship with marijuana related to artistic endeavors is: it's like the jumper cables for the battery in your car. OK, sometimes you just want to tune out and relax, but sometimes you have some marijuana and it's like you just put the spark in the battery. Now that your engine's running, you believe you're in a creative mood that wouldn't have happened if you hadn't smoked. And then you say, "Wow, I like this!" And then tomorrow you smoke again, 'cause you think, "Oh, the same thing's gonna happen again," but what's actually happening is that now you're taking what was actually just a spark and you're trying to treat it like it's the gasoline.

Weed can never be the gasoline that runs your engine. It could be the spark that turns the battery on, but everything else is *you*. Sometimes it turns on the systems that prime you to get back into a different focus, but you can't rely on it to keep you in that state, and the minute that you find yourself looking at it that way every day, then it's no longer the thing that it was that got you in that direction. At that point it's a crutch.

JW: I think that makes a lot of sense. In my research and in some of the conversations I've had, I've learned about people who, for example, want to write a song or a poem, so they smoke and it just comes to them. To them, the weed made the song happen, but I wonder if the song was already there, and smoking was more about self-conditioning and setting aside specific time and intention for art making. Is it causal, or is it correlated?

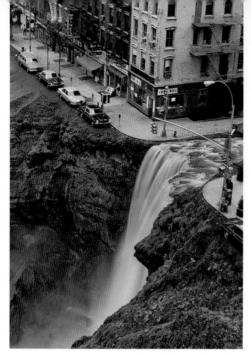

Urban Falls

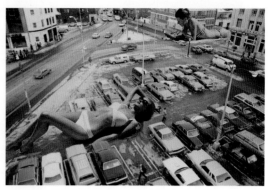

Beech Streets

GS: There's something to be envied in that ability. That could very well be the truth, that they smoke and then they're in that space, but that's not how it works for me. If you're not in a creative spirit, and then one day you smoke some weed, and you get into a creative spirit, you might smoke weed every single day, thinking you're sustaining it. But the funny thing is, the minute you stop smoking it, your mind clears up, and not being high is the new way to think differently. The thing that sparked your creativity was the change in your mentality.

JW: Like an overall state change.

GS: Exactly. It's a state change. Once you change that state, things have a different perspective, and when things have a different perspective, whatever your normal habits or coping mechanisms are, they no longer mean anything because they no longer have that power over you for the moment. You're on this mental highway, and it could take you to good places, but just like all road trips, you can enjoy the scenery, but at a certain point, you think, "Are we there yet?" And then you get out of the car, and it's better to be out of the car. That's sort of like what it's like for me. I wanna go on the road trip. But after so many miles, being out of the car is more interesting.

JW: Are there other types of state changes that you use to get creative?

GS: The most important state change that is always effective, even on a bad day, is exercise. And I mean, hardcore exercise. Some people, if their phone is gonna die and they don't have a charger, it's like the world is gonna end. For me, if I don't exercise at least four times a week, then that's when the panic sets in. It's that important to my mental and physical health. Exercise puts me in a primed state. I feel like I'm clearer. I hate to sound like one of these people that goes into a high school auditorium and says, "Get high on life!" You know what I mean? But it's true. Get your blood flowing. Work out, listen to some Daft Punk, and go for it. And then when you get out of the gym, you're more excited for things than when you went in.

Sometimes I don't wanna be clear, and that's when weed is useful, but in that case, weed is a helpful distraction. I think a lot of times people turn to things that are going to distract them from the discomfort of their lives.

JW: Do you think that discomfort is important for development as a creative?

GS: Yes and no. If you're a painter, you need your paint, you need your studio, and you need the light to come in a certain way. There are certain conditions that have to be right. So you might be someone who wants to embrace the chaos of life. You could be Jack Kerouac and go on an adventure, but Jack Kerouac wrote *On the Road* after the adventure was over, sitting at a typewriter in a comfortable room, where he could have tea and candles or whatever. Comfort is very important. You need the roof over your head, you need the pen and the paper, and you need the distractions tuned out to achieve a certain amount of focus. All of that can only be achieved in a stable, comfortable environment. I do believe that discomfort is extremely important, but I also know that if you are constantly in a corner, worried about rent or actual matters of life, then you just don't have the luxury of focus, and focus is extremely important. Focus really can only be achieved, I think, in a place of serenity and comfort.

JW: So when you choose to smoke, what is it that drives you to make that decision?

GS: Sometimes, I'll just feel like smoking some weed. It's not like food where I've gotta eat. It's strange. It is an impulse, I guess, but I've also had that impulse and then decided not to smoke. There's no rhyme or reason. My relationship with it is so passive, and the only time I'm ever very serious about smoking marijuana is when I'm serious about *not* smoking it. I never get serious about *having* to smoke. Sometimes I will want that jump start, so I smoke, but I'm always very careful about not letting it become this thing that I need. There are chapters of my life where I'm gonna smoke more weed. In those chapters, I'm glad that I have marijuana in my life. It's not an all-the-time go-to, but I'm happy it's there, the same way that I'm happy that I have jumper cables in my car.

Anna Pollock

visual artist

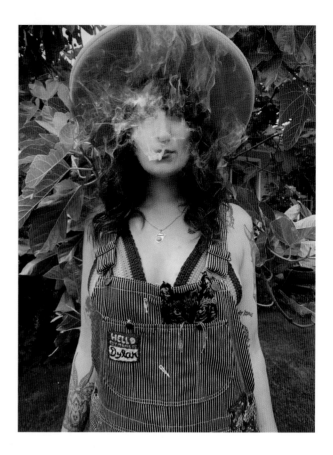

Anna Pollock's art evokes the color and energy of a different time. With hard-edged borders and blocks of bold, arresting color, the posters and album art she creates for musical acts and performers exude a musicality of their own. In color palettes and sensibilities that harken back to the golden era of musical posters created by genre-defining artists like Peter Max and Victor Moscoso, Pollock's work feels familiar and yet absolutely original. There's something very melodic about the way she combines text and imagery in a cohesive composition. You find yourself wanting to explore every square inch of the pieces she designs, as if each stroke or line will lead you somewhere exciting.

Born and raised in the Pacific Northwest on one of the islands near Seattle, she found her creative energy at a young age. With a directive from her parents to either create art or go outside and explore, Pollock formed an identity around the values of personal exploration and artistic expression. Through high school and college, she studied visual arts but always felt a deep connection to music. Around that same time, she found a place in her life for cannabis and started to develop a creative process that incorporated all three interests.

Sitting in a cozy, softly lit room, she smiles as she reflects on a lifelong dream to be a musician, but with a true talent for visual arts and a self-proclaimed lack of musical skill, she manages to find the best of both worlds in her work. When combining cannabis and music, Pollock feels transported and inspired. She explains, "When I smoke, it's like

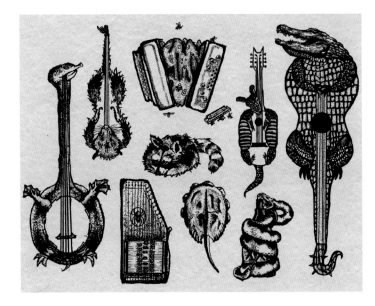

the floodgates are open and it expands my creative thinking." Music gives her an almost synesthetic experience where sounds appear visually, helping her formulate new ideas and imagined worlds to sketch and paint.

A summer in New York City provided a formative introduction to other artists and new experiences, when Pollock attended a painting workshop there as a teenager. On an outing to Central Park with some of the other students, an older kid bought some pot for the group, and her creative flow immediately expanded. "I was a pretty uptight kid," she explains, "so it loosened me up a lot and also made me realize that not everything I had been taught was real."

Growing up like many American teens in her generation, Pollock received a Reagan-inspired anti-drug education in school. "I never thought I could use pot and be a productive member of society," she explains, but with a new outlook on the potential positives of cannabis use and her ability to push past internal roadblocks, she was inspired. "I feel like I can only go one route when I'm not high. My brain will follow a very structured path." But after she smokes "it's like a total immersion into this very warm, protective, creative space. You can really just forget about everything else. I found this really good, sweet spot where I work with it, and it works with me, and I'm able to do what I want and do it happily."

Finding and calibrating her ideal creative process took time. "When I first started smoking, it was pretty overwhelming: the rush of images and ideas and tangents. But I learned how to focus it to expand my creative thinking," she tells me. With added focus from smoking, Pollock has more energy to work through iterations of her ideas and designs. She sometimes spends long, continuous periods of time on a piece. "I'll go over it in detail," she explains with a determined look in her eye, "I can get into it for a whole day. It's a state of being. I go into a meditative mindset, and I lose total track of everything else. It's blank. Everything's intentional, but you're also blank."

Pollock considers herself lucky to have found a direction with her work that allows her to thrive both professionally and artistically. Although she's trained in oil painting and considers it her first love, Pollock's current process involves sketching on paper and then transferring her ideas to her digital tablet. It's a process that she can easily utilize at home or wherever she happens to be when the inspiration takes her. Digital work allows her to adjust as needed and have more of a sense of fluidity as she creates.

To get in the right mindset for her work, Pollock likes to smoke, put on some music, and dance a bit to loosen up, she tells me, slowly shimmying her shoulders for effect. Then, once

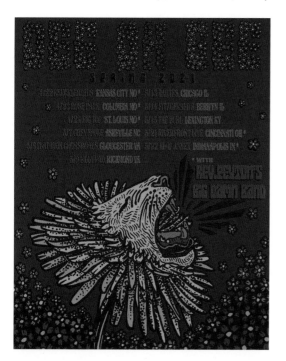

she's in the right mood, "I'll just settle in and just jam and draw." Without cannabis, she explains "I can produce some cool work, but I never want to look at it again because of the energy and how it makes me feel." For her, that work represents creation outside of her comfort zone, arrested by self-judgement and overthinking. Creation, she believes, should inhabit the world of free-flowing self-expression, rather than self-criticism.

Her personal process works. Musicians and their fans are incredibly positive about Pollock's work, and she attributes much of that satisfaction and success to her uninhibited creative methods. With the

CANNABIS FOR CREATIVES

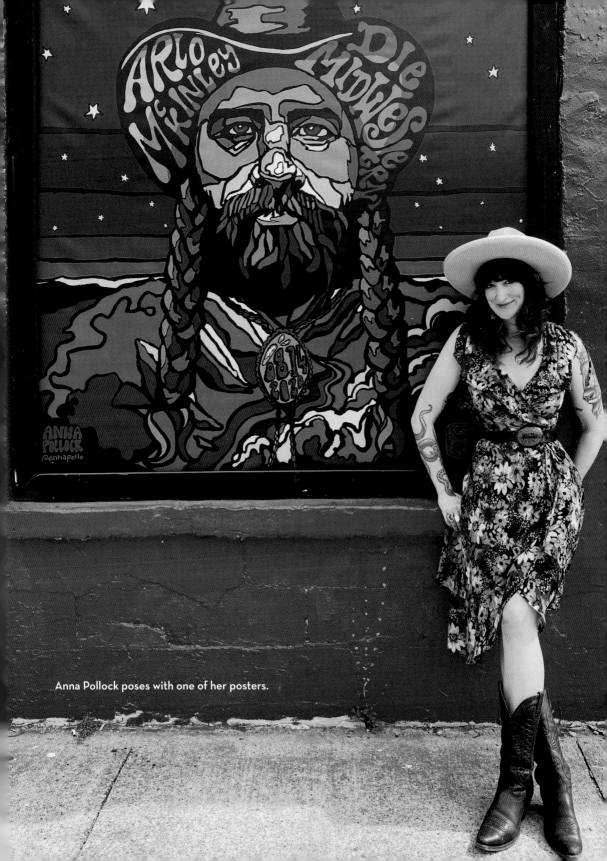

Anna Pollock poses with one of her posters.

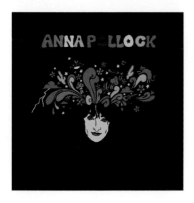

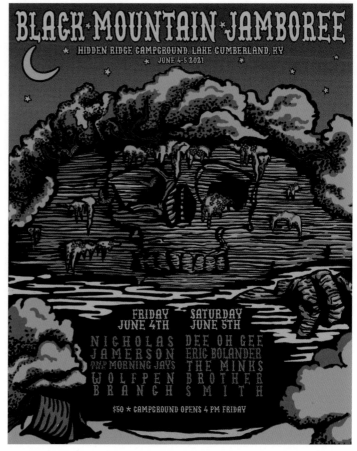

influx of new commissions and introductions to widening networks of musicians, Pollock feels like she's more connected to creative people than ever before, and it's inspired her to continue along her path of experimentation.

Recently, at the suggestion of her doctor, Pollock started microdosing with mushrooms for anxiety management as well as other health benefits. She finds that the psilocybin combined with cannabis have had positive therapeutic results for her frame of mind, both personally and creatively. "It's interesting to reacquaint myself with these plants as tools and medicines. I'm reprogramming my brain to see these as helpful things and not scary things."

Reeducating herself on the Nixon–Reagan eras of drug control and how it has affected multigenerational consciousness about psychoactive substances, has become an important pursuit for her. Over the years, she's received some criticism about the potential dangers of

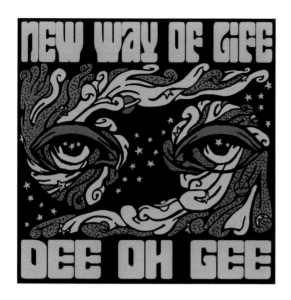

her cannabis use from a few people in her life. "It's been very interesting to see them be so steadfast in believing that marijuana and mushrooms are evil tools and then turn around and take pain pills that their doctor prescribes. Pharmaceuticals can be a really great benefit to a lot of people, but to think that something created in a lab is healthier than something that doesn't have x, y, and z side effects, and also comes from the earth is an interesting take. It's what I believed for a while too," she adds, "It's what we grew up learning."

The artistic community tends to be more open to her frame of mind. "My noncreative friends definitely see it as a crutch at times, whereas my friends who are musicians…they're the same as me. We feel like cannabis and creativity are so interlinked."

Living in Washington, a state where adult use of marijuana is legal and the decriminalization of mushrooms appears to be on the horizon, Pollock feels fortunate to have had the access and freedom she enjoys. She can purchase her ideal strains in a dispensary. Forbidden Fruit is a favorite, as is Elon Musky, which provides the greatest creative high she's ever had. Pollock prefers joints to concentrates or dabs, but she also enjoys edibles for when she needs to be more discreet. At times, vaping gives Pollock the wrong type of high for making art, but if any high comes on too strong, music brings her back. She cultivates an environment filled with comforting music and tries to direct her energy in a positive direction. "If I'm too high, my mind is racing. I just let it race and try to steer it somewhere in the direction of what I'm doing and see if I can get an overflow of ideas." In her heightened flow state, she attempts to lock on to one of her tangents and let it carry her to a place of productivity.

Cannabis, Pollock explains, "makes me far more able to enjoy living in the moment, enjoy my surroundings, enjoy the music that's playing, enjoy the food." She smiles, and her eyes widen. "I think about all the things that I normally wouldn't be able to do. The colors are bright; everything's cheerful and happy. Weed helps me access the fantasy that I'm trying to create."

Nelson Ruger

visual artist and designer

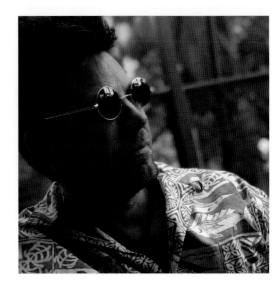

I've known Nelson Ruger for most of my
adult life. He not only introduced me
to my husband, but he also served as
a significant creative influence and mentor when I was developing as an artist myself. He
demonstrated that creativity and art can positively impact people's lives, from the audiences
viewing the work, to the artists themselves.

Having transitioned through multiple creative careers, from theatrical design and production
management, to serving as the creative director for a theme park, he now finds success
and fulfillment through painting and digital design. In his current work, he draws from his
theatrical background and experience to evoke mood and wonder. His art makes people feel
things. He also designed the cover of this book.

JW: Can you give me a little background on your artistic journey?

NELSON RUGER: I went into theatrical design because I liked painting with light and
scenery and creating three-dimensional worlds on stage. I really enjoyed the reactions
that my work got from people. They always remarked how good the lighting made them
feel or how the scenery evoked feelings in them that they welcomed.... And then theatre
ate my soul. And by that, I mean it just worked me to death, and I decided it wasn't worth
it anymore. I went to work in retail briefly, and only working a 40-hour week allowed me
to actually get into painting. I like how the work makes people feel. I like being able to
bring the feelings of awe, wonder, and "Wow, that's damn cool and makes me feel good"
to people's lives on a regular basis.

JW: When did cannabis come into your life?

NR: I tried it when I was in college because that's what college is there for. It was in a social environment, and it did nothing. Everybody else was just really, really high, and whenever you're in a situation like that, it's a little weird. You feel left out. It was weird enough that I didn't really ever want to do it again. I'd be fine with going to parties with it, but I didn't really want to try it again, just because I felt so ostracized by my own brain and body.

Then, all the systems and processes that I had put in place to handle my ADD started to fail, and because my headspace was getting more and more difficult to manage, the weed started to work a little bit more. I remember a time in your apartment when smoking worked, and I was like, "You have got to be kidding me!"

Almost a year ago, I'd been formally diagnosed with high-functioning ADD, and it was taking a real toll on my mind and body and spirit. I was having a hard time managing all the stuff that was going on, and I was doing business meetings and it had been a really rough day. I got back to my hotel and called for a cannabis delivery, and it was just instant calm, followed by focus, and the ability to actually breathe and let go of all the noise. It was like somebody just flipped a switch in my head. And after that, weed became my number-one anxiety management tool and go-to when I'm way too obsessive–compulsive about something. It allows me to step back and breathe a little bit.

JW: Do you think it makes you more creative?

NR: Yes, absolutely. In a little bit of a different way. Weed allows me to relax, get into the actual creative zone where ideas flow, and just let everything happen. I remember one project recently where I was doodling on my iPad just trying to get something going, and it really wasn't working. I got high, and it allowed the ideas that were in my head to come forward. It was funny because I remember struggling and struggling and struggling and struggling

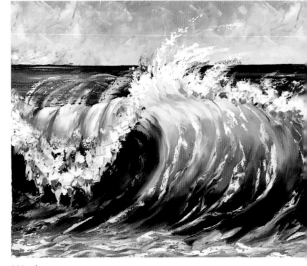

Windswept

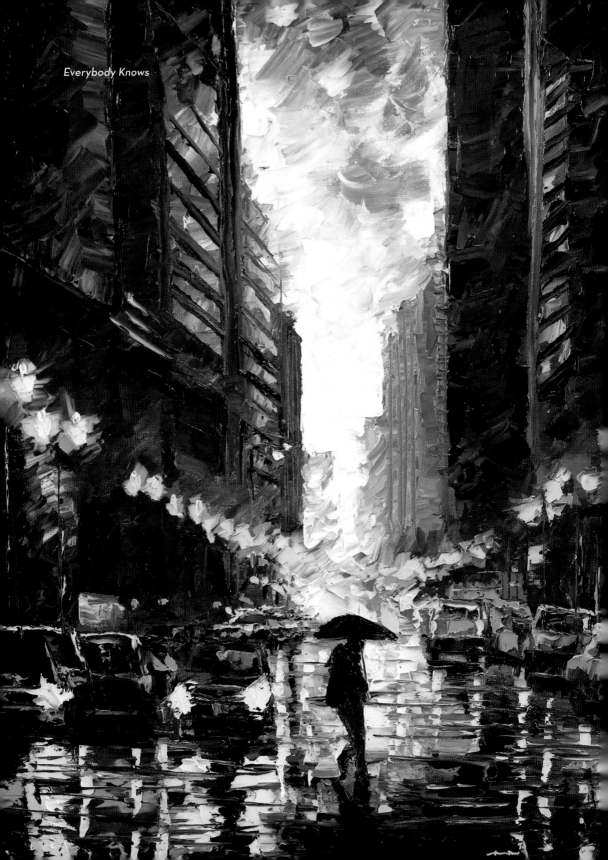

Everybody Knows

and struggling, and then getting high, and then the concept was in, and it was done. It just opens the floodgates.

JW: What other parts of your process are there? What's the start to finish?

NR: So I'm a super technical guy. I actually enjoy the technical part of the process as much as I enjoy the creative part of the process. I'll create a foundation of what I'm going for with my iPad. When I start into the actual physical part, I do all the line drawings and stuff, and I transfer that to a canvas. Then I'll block in all the major colors with acrylic. After that is when the actual fluid creative process happens with paint. It's like you're making magic on top of this illustration, and it's adding all of the cool bits that make people go, "Oh, wow, look at that," or make people feel a certain way.

JW: To use a music analogy, it sounds like you mark out what the melody is going to be, and then the really creative part starts when you can figure out the harmonies and all the intricacies.

NR: Yeah, and that's where I prefer to have weed nearby, so it turns into a creative process and not an obsessive-compulsive process. I will say though, weed can sort of dilate time, and time sort of expands on its own to where it'll go from something that I work on over an afternoon, to something I work on for days.

JW: How do you know when you're finished?

NR: Someone usually has to say to me, "It's time to walk away," 'cause I won't know. It's a difficult thing, and sometimes I won't listen and I'll go back and touch the canvas. It's a running joke: "It's done. Until tomorrow." Somebody usually has to tell me to stop touching the damn thing.

JW: Do you think that comes from your foundation in theatre, and the fact that there was always an end point where the show opens, and you can't really mess with it anymore, and you don't have that with a painting?

NR: Yeah, that's why I ask other people. It's like I'm finally opening the curtain and people go, "Hey, you're out of previews."

JW: Why do you think cannabis makes you more creative?

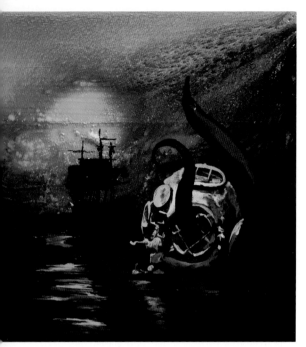

Anybody Seen Bob

NR: It's getting me out of the trenches and back up to 50,000 feet where I can see the big picture and stay there until I find the thing that I wanna zero in on. When I'm in the trenches, I don't know what I really should be focusing on.

JW: What does it feel like when you've smoked?

NR: The little things and the little mistakes don't matter, because now I know how to fix everything, and I know that almost nothing is unfixable. Without weed, I don't know that all the time.

JW: So it softens your inner critic a little bit?

NR: That's a good way to put it. Yeah, absolutely. 'Cause it does allow me to go, "Alright, that sucks," but I can walk away and come back to it tomorrow. If I haven't smoked, you'll need the Jaws of Life to get me out of there. It's brutal. It does help me to step back a little bit, and I always know that it's time to step back when somebody hands me the vape.

JW: Do you gravitate toward any specific varieties or strains?

NR: I've got a sativa for during the day and indica for night. I have an indica vape by my bed that is just for going to sleep, 'cause it will take me to happy, dreamlike places. There are a lot of times I can't sleep at night anymore, and it allows me to go to a really, really good place, and sometimes a really creative place that I can wake up and take with me, whereas the sativas really allow me to just dial back my daytime stress and zone in and be creative.

JW: Are there other creative pathways you're employing to get in the zone?

NR: Absolutely. So meditation is one; fitness is another one. Running and going to the gym really help me get zoned in. Keeping my space clean is also really important to me because if my worktable is just a mass of brushes and paint, I can't see anything if I need it. I have also discovered that the ritual of making a drink, not even drinking it sometimes, but just making a drink makes me feel good. It relaxes me. Going over to the bar and picking the different ingredients and mixing them together—just the simple act of making a stupid margarita, or even a margarita with no booze in it, will help me to get back in a really good place. Ultimately, what I want my art to do is either send you on an adventure or send you on a vacation, it's one of the two, and making a drink sort of embodies both for me.

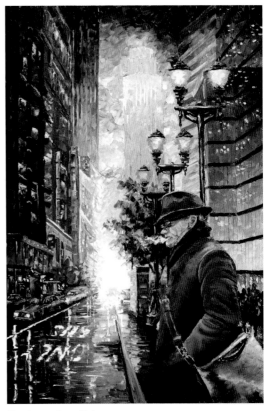

For Immediate Release

JW: How does your creative process change if you don't have access to pot?

NR: I'm a complete asshole! Not always. Once I'm in the zone, I'm usually pretty good, but otherwise I get lost in all the crap, and then I just get mean, and surly, and I'm an unpleasant person to be around, as opposed to when I'm on weed and I'm just like, "Hey, let's make some beautiful shit that makes people happy" and I'm evoking those feelings into the canvas.

JW: Can you tell me about creating the cover for this book?

NR: I was going through a lot of Covid stuff at the time, and I was reaching my wits' end. Creatively, I was finding myself feeling really boxed in. I kept gravitating away from the things that I wanted to gravitate toward. I couldn't get near it. My brain would block it out and pretend like it wasn't there. I remember asking myself, "Why am I gravitating away from that? What is so scary about that?" And I remember feeling like there's so much literal joy waiting to happen in the creative process of it and in the idea of this amazing fantasy world where anything you wanna create is totally possible if I just loosen up and relax and let the process happen.

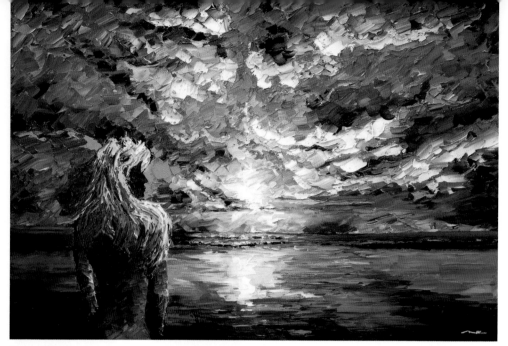

Sirens Dreams

I remember getting high and being on my iPad all night, stoned and relaxed and just letting the ideas happen. So much of it was just throwing stuff on the screen and seeing what happened. It only took an hour before I found it. It felt like it was full of creative joy, and I was soaking myself in it, both through smoking and through allowing myself to have that much of a beautiful, joyful creative process.

JW: It's just so cool. It's everything I ever wanted for the cover.

NR: It was such a fun project and so full of joy.

JW: Are there any other cannabis insights you want to share?

NR: I just wish I'd been introduced to it so much earlier in a really healthy and humane way without any of the bullshit societal issues that surround it, because now that I'm using it regularly, I can't imagine how much of my life would have been better. It allows me to loosen up. As I'm going through life, I'm finding that the quality of your experience is far more important than the quality of the stuff around you, and more of that experience becomes accessible when you're not hanging on so tight. Some people can do that through meditation, and that's enough. Some of us do things that are really crazy and intense and push us beyond our limits, and we need a way to be able to manage that. It makes a really big difference.

Nathaniel C. Hunter
author and activist

Nathaniel C. Hunter (not his real name) has always felt an impulse toward creativity. Professionally, he directs that energy into writing nonfiction books and social activism. Trouble in his teenage years and young adulthood resulted in the absence of a healthy, supportive, and productive social circle. He turned to less than healthy coping mechanisms and outlets for his emotions. Although he'd always been a creative person, drawing, painting, writing, and performing music, it wasn't until his mid-20s that he found a relationship with cannabis and with society in general that could propel him forward in a positive direction.

Today, the benefits of cannabis come in many forms for Hunter. Psychologically, he explains, "it gives me the space to center myself. I've always been very introverted and shy, so pot has always felt protective, and it also felt directive, too, because it allowed me to shut out all the crazy stress that I've always surrounded myself with, to bring me back to who I was."

Though he doesn't smoke enough to feel high or impaired, he does smoke very regularly, an activity that has been exceedingly beneficial in his daily life. "It helps my focus—my productivity, my ability to interact with other people, my ability to actually dig into tasks and see them through to the end. A lot of things distract me. It takes the edge off to get rid of the noise." From a medicinal perspective, cannabis helps Hunter to thrive in his personal and professional life. When it's time to write a book, though, that's when he shakes things up to explore how cannabis can set a productive creative state in motion.

For Hunter, the best writing occurs in an isolated marathon of creativity. He travels to a natural location with legal cannabis, stops off at a dispensary to gather supplies, and then he works long hours, free from internet access, free from external distractions, and free to explore his thoughts and find inspiration. When he can connect to his creativity via cannabis, he says it feels like he's "alone in a world of wonder. Because I'm an introvert, it's important for me to recharge alone. On these retreats, cannabis forces me to be alone *within* myself

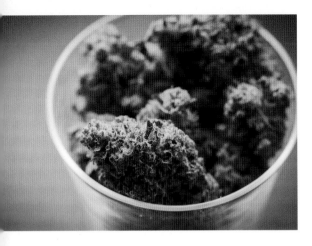

and not just be alone *by* myself. I've always been a big thinker, so it allows me to connect the dots between the ideas and the reality."

Choice of environment is important to the creative process as well. Hunter explains, "I usually find an outdoor, secluded space, whether it's a forest, or desert, or wherever. I take myself outside of the world physically and figuratively. I would go to rent a cabin in the middle of nowhere, sometimes it didn't have running water, sometimes it was a treehouse where the nearest resident wasn't for two miles. I even wrote on a houseboat in Amsterdam for a couple of weeks."

Other than eating meals (which he sometimes forgets to do) and sleeping (which happens very little during writing binges), Hunter focuses his energy on writing, whether it be stream of consciousness, or working closely within an outline. He makes sure that he always has the next joint handy so if he's on a roll creatively, he can keep going as his inspiration demands.

More subtle sativas are ideal for maintaining Hunter's sense of clarity, calm, and focus, without the feeling of impairment or any kind of body high. Even so, he always approaches editing with a completely clear head. "Sometimes what I write gets really dreamy. It sounds great when you're writing it, but it maybe doesn't make a whole lot of sense, or it's too wordy or flowery," he says. So when he gets back home, he reapproaches and refines his work.

Though smoking is an activity he always enjoys alone, he doesn't mind the company of others once he's reached a more lucid and outgoing state. Cannabis, in his experience, softens the edges of anxiety and depression, while focusing his mind and providing clarity, so he can live his life in a way that feels positive, productive, and enjoyable. In his history as a pot smoker, Hunter finds comfort in the increased inspiration. "I feel like I've had a million bright ideas, or bright sentences, or bright thoughts, acting as signposts saying 'Go in this direction.' These moments are the atoms that make the molecule."

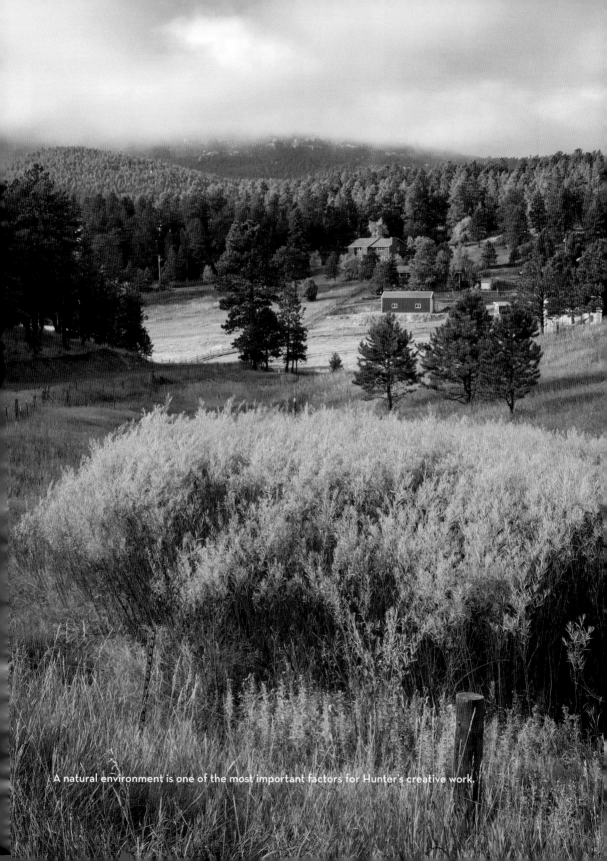

A natural environment is one of the most important factors for Hunter's creative work.

Kenton Williams

musician

Kenton Williams is a musician, songwriter, and performer who lives in New Jersey, but he is a New Yorker at heart. He fills his life with music and performance even while engaging in other passions professionally. Creativity and an impulse toward music have been two of the defining pursuits of his life.

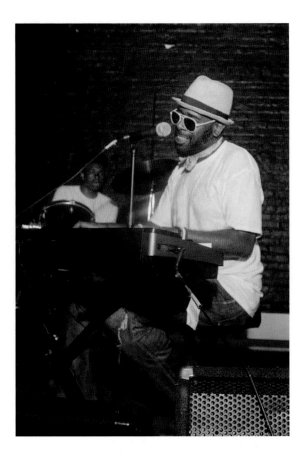

JW: Can you tell me a bit about who you are, what you do, and what your artistic journey has been?

KENTON WILLIAMS: I've been performing as The Ken Demitri Show for 15 years. I'm 41 now, and I have been a singer-songwriter since I was 13. I started acting when I got to college on a dare. That was also part of my journey because it melded into the artist that I became: an all-around performer. I incorporate a lot of comedy into my shows. I'm moderately funny, and so I do a lot of storytelling in between songs as part of the show package and all of that. I managed to not get famous by sleeping through a bunch of auditions in my 20s, 'cause I was high, and also I was very stubborn about my process and what I was trying to do as a rapper who sang. Everybody was just like, "Yeah, pick one, you gotta sing or you gotta rap." And I was like, "This is dumb. I'll just wait for you guys to all catch up." Eventually they did; by then, I was an old person.

JW: When did cannabis come into your life?

KW: I've smoked every day since I was 16, although, growing up in the hood in Brooklyn, I was around it all the time. When I was 13, the neighborhood system for cannabis distribution—I'm sanitizing this a little bit on purpose—emanated from the first floor of the building that I lived on the third floor of. And so a lot of us kids made a couple of bucks here or there, running packages up and down the street because it was inconspicuous. We were always being sent to the store anyway, so if you run this down the block, nobody's gonna suspect anything. You come back and keep two of the 25 dollars for yourself, and now you've got your snack for the day. Do that four times a week…now you've doubled your allowance, and nobody knows how. So I always knew what herb was. We came from these environments where cannabis culture—this is the way we talk about it now—was completely a part of all of our lives: adults, kids, everybody. It wasn't taboo. Granted, you didn't want your parents to know you smoked weed, but your parents smoked weed too.

JW: Do you have particular strains that are your favorite?

KW: Yeah, yes, you're asking specifically in terms of those funny names that we give everything? I've been a White Widow person ever since I found it for the first time when I was 22. It's still around, unlike most of the strains from back then. There's no finding Strawberry Haze that's actually Strawberry Haze in 2021. But White Widow still comes around, and I love it when I find it.

JW: Do you remember any kind of shift in perspective about it when you realized, "Alright, this isn't just for having fun with my friends," that it could be about feeling more creative?

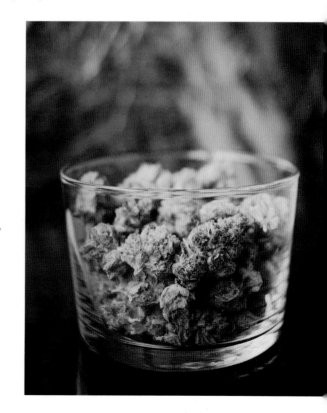

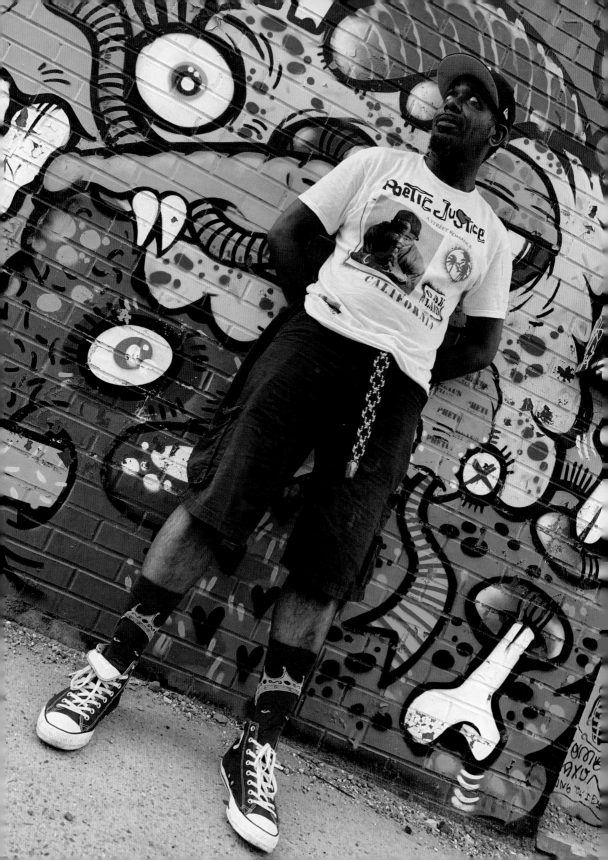

KW: When my friend taught me to rap. Because at first I wouldn't rap in front of anybody. I had been writing for years, but that's not the same thing as somebody teaching you the art form of crafting your raps. My friend, his rhyme schemes when we were in college were always so much more complex than half the shit guys that I knew were writing, and he was just coming off the top of his head with it. I needed to be in that space to keep up. My senior year, a lot of my smoking weed was tied up with making music. Those two social things went together in a way that they hadn't before, even though at 15, I would be up at 1:00 a.m. with headphones and the Casio writing songs after smoking a blunt in the backyard. But I wasn't consciously connecting them in the way that I began to do when I was 20 at school.

JW: Do you feel that pot is necessary for your creativity as far as writing or performing?

KW: I'm old now, so I don't smoke before I perform, or at least not with my rock and roll band, because I can't access the upper reaches of my register as easily. I am just not in the vocal shape to sing at the top of my register for an hour after I've smoked, even though physiologically for most of my career, smoking has always been part of my warmup because of the way that it opens your vocal passages. Because of the amount that I have smoked in my life, it's not like I'm gonna take two puffs and then I'm gonna go out there and be stoned and in the zone.... I would have to *smoke*. And so then if I do that, by the 35th minute of the show—which is just me, howling into this microphone 'cause it's a metal band—I just don't have it. And so I've had to figure that out.... But if it's a show where I get to sit in the corner and play the piano, and sing a bunch of background vocals, I smoke in the middle of that shit. I smoke on stage with a joint hanging out of my mouth.

JW: And what about smoking for writing?

KW: When it comes to day-to-day activities, and for me writing songs is a day-to-day activity like brushing my teeth, it's just this thing that I do. And so...Is it part of it? It's enough part of my life that you couldn't say it's not, but within that very same token, it's enough part of my life that it is not...It's not like, "Oh shit, I haven't smoked, I'm not coming up with any ideas." You know what I mean? But then there are no days that I don't smoke.

JW: OK, so it's like: how do you define where it begins and ends, because it's such a common thing throughout your life?

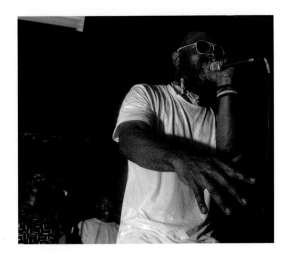

KW: Correct. I'm creative all the time. I think in rhyme. I literally process my thoughts in couplets or quartiles. I think in verse. It's who I am.

JW: What is your creative process when you intend to write?

KW: I don't intend to write, so it depends. There's the creation process, and then there's the practice process. All of my creation is spontaneous. I don't sit down to write. I used to. As I got better as a songwriter, I also got older and became more of a smoker. It became more of a thing in my life. To say that there's a point where I stopped getting high to get in the zone is a little bit difficult because, one might say, I *live* in that zone.

JW: What does it feel like to be in that zone, specifically when you're high?

KW: I've always smoked for the same reason, which is that there's too much going on inside my head. Smoking slows it down and allows me to have better access to pick and choose my thoughts and stay in a linear place with them. If I'm not stoned, my practice would be ineffective, but physically what it feels like, is very different at 41 than it was at 21, because I haven't had a body high in 10 years. I'm sure that's resistance, and I've built up a tolerance. If you wanna talk in the way that physiologically feels, it's like a headband.

JW: How does it feel like a headband?

KW: The ways that people typically use indica and sativa, those things are reversed for me. I don't particularly like indicas anymore because they're kind of useless in terms of what I am trying to do. While they relax my body, I don't really feel high in my body, and so what they do is just turn me into a potato while leaving my mind untouched. So now I'm just this sentient potato who's looking around at the world, and it's the worst. In my everyday life, all I want is this headband. And I'm using that to describe both the way it feels and also a representation of what it's actually doing to my head. It's putting some boundaries around where I'm allowing my mind to wander off to.

Nikki Barber

multidisciplinary artist

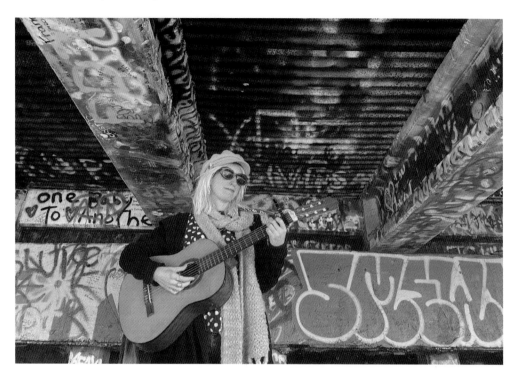

A sense of community has always been central to Nikki Barber's creative life. The vocalist and guitarist for The Minks, a Nashville-based "psychedelic-bloos" band, first set out for the Music City in the pursuit of building a community for herself around a common love for music. Less than 10 years later, Barber is the front woman for a much beloved band with a unique genre-bending sound, and she designs and fabricates unique pieces for her fashion line, Nikki Stitch.

Barber's home in East Nashville serves as her costume shop, personal recording studio, and creative sanctuary. From her eclectically decorated room, filled with important artifacts from her life, she sips tea and shares what she's learned about creativity.

A dabbler in many artistic pursuits, Barber views the act of creation as the common through line that guides her work, rather than any specific title or pigeonhole. She explains, "I don't really like to say that I'm only a musician or only a designer or anything. I'm an artist. I love to draw. I really love to take pictures. I love visual things. I always have five creative projects going at once, but that's just how my brain works."

An art-focused community center in her hometown of Gettysburg, PA, provided a nurturing backdrop for her early experiences with art, music, and collaboration during her formative teenage years. "As divine timing would have it," she tells me, "I happened to be there at the right time when there was a big group of artists my age doing things." By watching touring bands come through and perform, Barber and her peers discovered firsthand that there was more to music than playing in the school orchestra: a realization that inspired her to dream of a life in a rock and roll band.

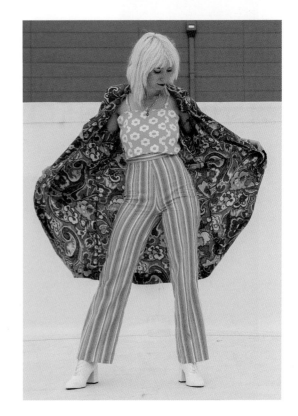

Although she studied fashion design in school, Barber eventually felt burned out by some of the more competitive and superficial aspects of the fashion industry and decided to pursue her creative goals on her own terms. Moving to Nashville provided a unique creative support system filled with equally ambitious and talented artists. As Barber began building her music career by writing songs, studying the guitar, and recording demos, she funded her pursuits by altering and designing stage costumes for other performers and musicians in her social circles. Through combined design and musical endeavors, she began to build the creative family that she now appreciates and relies upon for motivation, inspiration, and connection.

For Barber, creativity and community represent two of the three essential elements for artists. The third element—ideal for expansive vulnerability, inspiration, and confidence—is cannabis. She appreciates the things that pot has allowed her to experience and discover along her

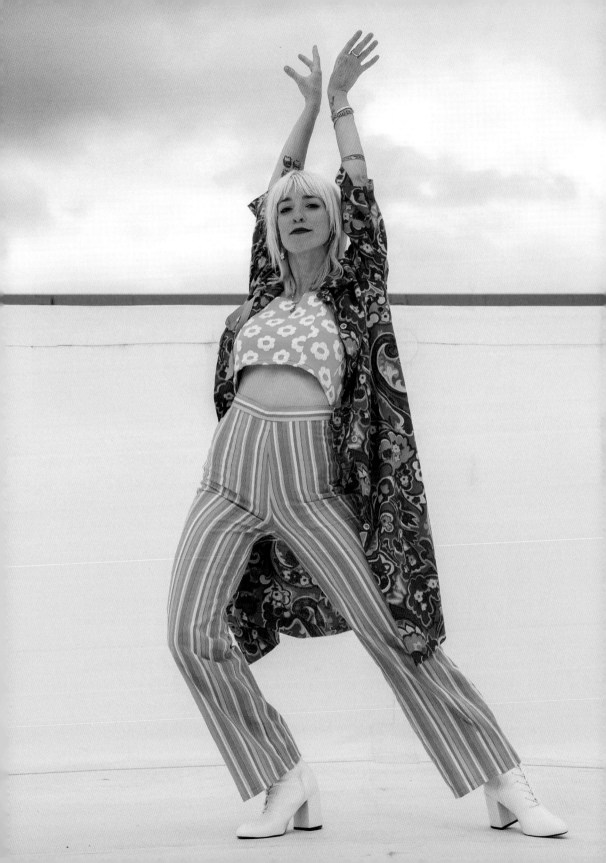

journey. "It's nice because it lets you sit in the moment a little more without thinking too much. If I'm about to play, it helps me prepare and it just enhances everything."

She first found an appreciation for cannabis in high school, around the same time she was forming early conclusions about her ambitions as an artist. Although she's been enjoying pot's effects fairly consistently since then, she's careful not to assign it too much significance in her process. "I don't want to use it as a crutch and think 'Oh, I need this to be creative,' but I do find that, especially when I'm by myself, it allows me to open up my brain a bit and free write or play things that I wouldn't necessarily think of otherwise. It opens up the boundaries."

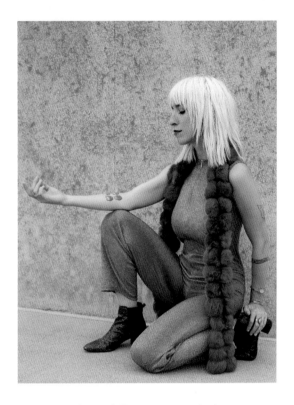

Cannabis also helps form new and stronger connections with her fellow artists. "I think it is a community thing for me. That's always been my favorite part about it, taking the time to sit together and enjoy a joint or whatever we have. We're also talking and growing together. It's nice to know you're all on the same level together, but even if one of us doesn't smoke, it's not like they're missing out or are estranged from the rest of us. They're still obviously part of the community."

For her solo creative sessions, working on a project or writing a song, Barber carefully curates her creative environment to get in the mood. Behind her sits what she refers to as her "altar," which serves as the centerpiece of her creative space. Surrounded by glowing Christmas lights, photos, postcards, colorful glass bottles, incense, and a Himalayan salt lamp, Barber feels creatively nurtured. Some of these items are so important to her sense of peace and comfort that she brings them along on the road when The Minks go on tour. She tells me, "I'm able to make any place my home if I have a few certain things that I love." With an environment of comfort, some jazz music in the background, and a smoke session with a one hitter or a joint, Barber finds a little something extra to help her engage in new ideas.

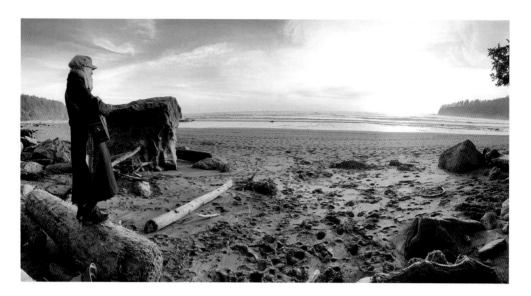

"I think it definitely enhances creativity for me, and I enjoy it. I really like it for dealing with anxiety and calming my emotions, which aids in allowing me to be more creative. I'm in that calm space from cannabis. As a daily thing, I don't like to be very blazed. I like a little hum in the back of my brain. That's where I think and feel the best with it." That little hum helped Barber conceive and pen the lyrics that became The Minks' second single, "I'm Okay," on their debut album "Light & Sweet."

While she generally prefers the qualities of an edible high, smoking is her go-to when preparing for a performance. "It depends on the strain, but when I smoke it's more of a head high, whereas when I ingest it, I feel it way more in my body as a physical relaxer. I like that feeling, but it does lay you down a little more. We play rock and roll, so we're playing pretty high-energy stuff. I'm already a pretty mellow person, so I don't need to add to my mellowness on the stage."

That she's secretly a mellow person is one of the more impressive things about Barber. The persona she embodies on stage and in The Minks' music videos is all sass, confidence, and high-energy charm. Both the way she carries herself and the aesthetic of the band's videos, album covers, and poster art, embody an energetic, driving, and timeless quality. She manages to simultaneously inhabit contemporary music and follow in the tradition of bands like Cream, Jefferson Airplane, and The Velvet Underground. Nikki Barber is a force, and she doesn't seem to be slowing down regardless of what circumstances get thrown her way.

After The Minks' East Coast tour in early 2020 was cut short by a series of cascading show cancellations and concerns about safety due to Covid-19, Barber, like many musicians, returned home to figure out how to keep herself busy, artistically motivated, and able to support herself. At first, fashion and clothing alteration projects drew her focus, but once it was clear that live music wasn't returning any time soon, Barber and her bandmates also found ways to keep writing, keep creating, and keep preparing for what would come next. "Once we started wrapping our heads around it, we were able to use the time wisely. We just finished recording a new album."

Much of her vital Nashville community has also been able to use the downtime of quarantine to create. It's something she views as an unexpected bonus of a complex and difficult situation. "It's funny, I had a bonfire with some friends last night. It was the first time I'd seen anybody in a really long time, and we just went around the fire, and everyone played their new demos and songs. I feel like we're all still processing, so it's taken a while for songs to come out of it, because it's such a new feeling for everybody. It's not an easy love song to write about. It's this vast emotional thing that we're still unpacking. I'm super excited for all the stuff that's going to come out of this. It's one silver lining."

With two completed albums, lots of rescheduled performances on the horizon, and a reinvigorated desire to perform in-person, live music again, Barber is ready for the next phase in her career. One thing that she doesn't anticipate changing any time soon is the position that cannabis has held in her life for some time. "It's definitely part of the culture I live in. I think as artists we're always trying to open our minds in some way to get to that next level or dimension. That's what we're always striving for. That's why we're typically never satisfied because we always think, 'Well I did this, but I need to go further.' I think that's why marijuana and drugs as a whole are typically more accepted within an artistic community, because we're striving to open these doors that haven't been opened before and to expand and see where it takes us."

Thanks to a solid and supportive community, cannabis to help her access her creativity, and some serious talent and drive, it seems like every door will open to Barber as soon as she arrives.

I'M OKAY

Composed by Nikki Barber (BMI) // Vocals and rhythm guitar by Nikki Barber // Bass, organ, and acoustic guitar by Joe Bisirri // Lead guitar by Ron Gallo // Drums and percussion by Dylan Sevey // Piano by Dylan Whitlow

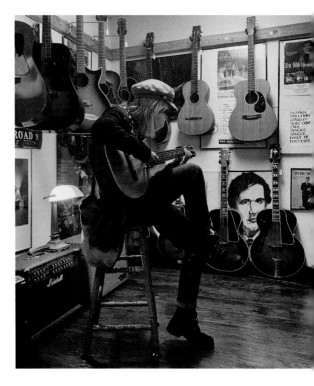

Well sister said to John, what the hell is
  going on? And all he did was turn up
  the sound.
He had no heart to tell her that gold is
  just burnt yellow, and what's lost can't
  always be found.
Sometimes I lose my mind, and all's I
  needs a sign to know I'm walking in the
  right way.
But I won't fear the dark, cuz I can feel the
  spark of creation making a perfect day.
Sometimes I get to feeling blue
But you know I'm gonna make it through
Cuz I'm okay.
I'm alright.
I'm feeling just groovy.
I'm okay.
Well I haven't had a lot to say for some
  days, cuz all my thoughts are visions
  of you.
You take my breathe away and make me
  feel okay, keep my head straight and my
  eyes see the truth.
Sometimes you meet a man who's figured
  out the plans, and makes you sure in what
  you believe.

He says, child don't lose your shine.
  Just keep having a good time. Keep
  your voice loud and your heart on
  your sleeve.
Well not everything is right, and I always
  gotta fight between my bleeding heart
  and my aching head.
But if I wake with a smile that can carry me
  for miles, I can twist and shout until I
  fall dead.
We're growing up so fast, but don't you
  dare look back cuz regrets will turn you
  to stone.
All of the mistakes help to appreciate the
  sweet taste of being thrown a bone.

Dope Chief

visual artist

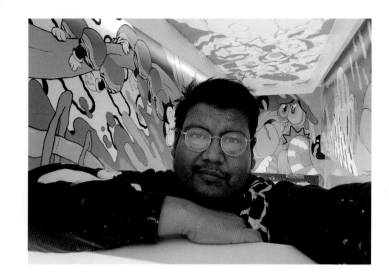

"Scale and medium. I tell artists that if you ever hit a mental or creative roadblock and you don't know how to get past it, two things that will always help you are changing the scale of your work and changing your medium."

Richard Campos Magarin, who works professionally under the name Dope Chief, has hit plenty of roadblocks in his career as an artist, but he's always found a way back to art that excites and inspires him.

"People who get into creative roadblocks," he continues, "have usually nailed down their formula so well that it's just that: a formula. When you get so good at something, where do you go? You're at the top of the mountain, and your brain gets bored. Things that create new challenges are great motivators for artists. We need things that push us back to where we're no longer a master of what we're doing." In his experience, those types of motivators force the creative mind into finding new methods and solutions. Whether you're a chef or a photographer or any other kind of artist, it's a way to shake things up.

In his studio in Hamilton, Ontario, Dope Chief sits in front of an electric pink wall—one of the signature colors in his work—and shares some of the insights he's learned since becoming a professional artist.

Dope Chief's art is brightly hued and energetic. With bold, curved lines, and an eye-catching aesthetic, his work draws on a love of illustration and the stylistic influences of 1930s to 1940s era cartoons.

"Growing up with Disney on VHS, I rewatched those tapes over and over until my mind melted. All of those things became influences for me." He loved drawing cartoons as a child, but as he got older, his interests changed to more adult themes. Dope Chief explains, "I've found it really interesting to combine and juxtapose this adolescent, very innocent format of cartoons with adult subject matter like sexuality, life, and death." He finds that heavier themes become more approachable when presented in the familiar, comfortable package of cartoons and a playful color palette: 1990s-esque neon pinks, purples, yellows, and teals are not only attention grabbing but soothing in a Nickelodeon-nostalgia kind of way.

In just a few minutes of talking to Dope Chief, it's obvious that he values thoughtful decision-making and strategy for every step in both his career and his creative process. Nothing happens by chance. When taking the leap to become a full-time artist, he wanted to be certain that each decision he made would lead him in the right direction toward his goals.

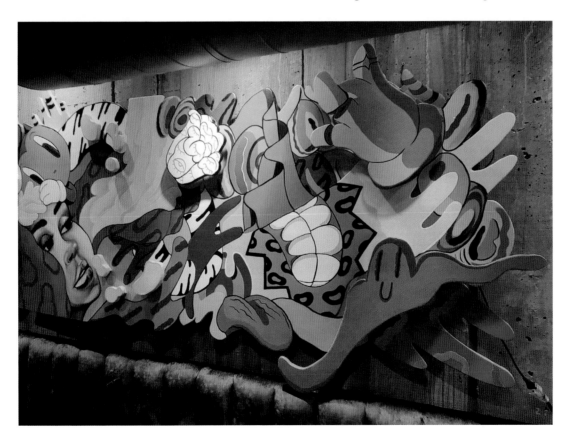

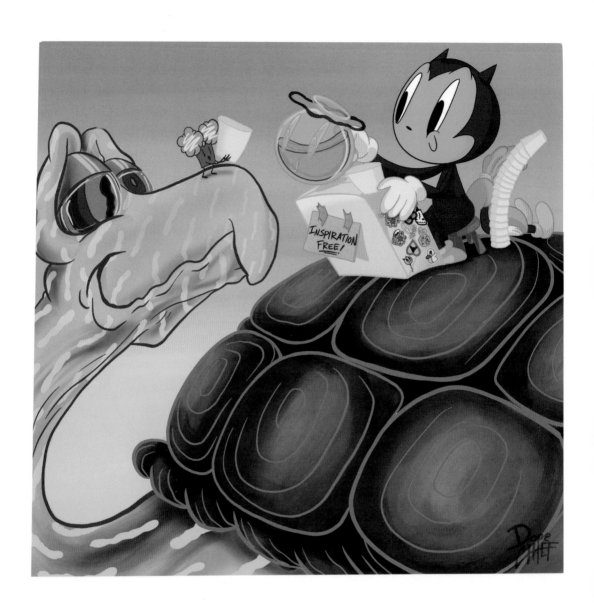

To make the best use of his time, some project work is delegated to his assistants. When creating large-format art installations, he outsources aspects like woodworking to allow him to focus on the overall vision and execution of the finished product. He believes that "If there are things you can outsource, no matter what business you're in, then outsource them. If there are jobs that other people can do, let them, because your time is going to be more valuable wherever your skill set is."

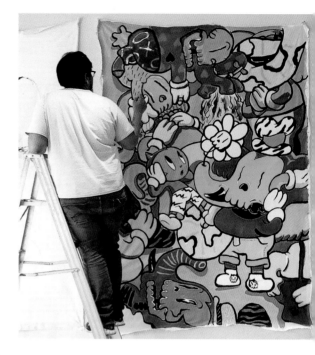

Ever analytical and self-reflective, Dope Chief has carefully honed the role that other influences play in his creative process. Anything from the act of procrastinating to the act of smoking a joint has its own carefully determined time and place. He believes that although procrastination may feel like time wasting and lead to self-judgement, it can be an important step in ideation.

"I'll procrastinate on a project for a month even though the actual work time would just be two or three days. At first, I think 'What if I wasn't this way? What if I could just do these things immediately? I'd be so much more efficient.' But is procrastination something that's actually inherent to my creative process? It allows me to keep thinking about a project and doing a lot of the mental work. Maybe I need that time to figure out how it's going to work in my head before I can do it in the physical world." It's an idea that, for any self-judging procrastinator, certainly sounds reassuring.

When the time comes to push through procrastination and jump-start the act of doing, Dope Chief finds that a joint can be a good motivator. The important distinction for his work is that creativity doesn't reside in cannabis, but smoking does help him sit down and achieve despite any motivational or mental blocks that he might have been experiencing.

"I have these moments of absolute frustration and fatigue. It feels like I can't focus. I can't bring myself to just sit down and work. I've given up so much: stability, proper income…I've

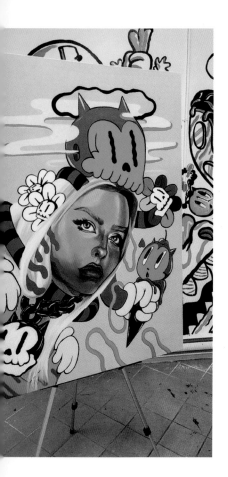

given everything I can to my art, so I find it frustrating to be in a position where I have the environment to create and still not be able to." That's where cannabis is most valuable to his workflow. He tells me, "My relationship with cannabis is like the starting of an engine. It says, 'Shut up. Just shut up and start.' Then nothing else matters because once I'm in that zone, I'm going. It's the thing that allows me the headspace where I can stop thinking and just explore."

Despite Dope Chief's appreciation for the motivation it can provide, he is wary of allowing cannabis to take on too prominent a position in his process. For concepting and interacting with commission clients, he values a clear head and being in control. "I don't want to rely on any external factor for creativity," he explains. Reflecting on the creative pursuits of his childhood, he realized that if he was capable of finding creativity organically back then, he should be able to access it just as easily now. The last thing he wants is to rely on pot for the inspiration of *what* to create. He's far more comfortable with cannabis as the initial push to get started.

Because he values that motivational, energetic aspect of smoking, sativas are Dope Chief's preference. He usually smokes a gram joint once or, at most, twice a day. He appreciates the positive qualities that cannabis can introduce, and although he's very transparent on social media about his pot use, he isn't looking to become a poster child for cannabis any time soon. "It's something I do, but I'm not interested in necessarily promoting it as something *everyone* should do to be more creative. I don't want people to assume that I revolve my life around it. It's something that you should respect. If someone asks me about it, I'm very honest, but I'm not on the campaign trail to see everyone smoking pot."

As he continues to grow and adapt as an artist, he enjoys pushing in new directions. Changing scale, like recent large-format installations, and changing medium, like an upcoming exploration into animation, is usually enough to inspire him creatively. But when he needs that extra push to get started, that's when he'll twist one up and get in the zone.

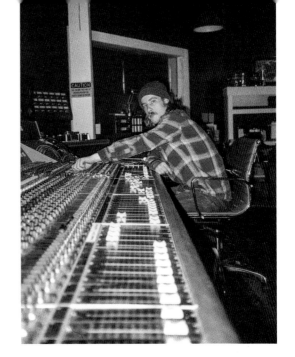

ARTIST INTERVIEW

Barrett Guzaldo

recording engineer
and musician

Barrett Guzaldo is a self-taught
recording engineer. He and
his business partner founded
Treehouse Records in 2014 on the
West Side of Chicago. They offer entirely analog recording services using vintage recording
equipment and have become an integral part of the Chicago music scene.

JW: How did you get into recording music?

BARRETT GUZALDO: I started learning guitar in middle school. I figured out how to play
and write songs, and I convinced all my friends to learn so we could get a band together. For a
while, it was just playing covers at a buddy's house. His dad used to be a musician back in the
day, so he got us the gear we needed to get started, including some recording equipment. I
was naturally drawn to recording, and I had test subjects to learn on and inspiration to acquire
this new skill. Eventually, I focused more on the engineering side. In high school, I got a studio
going in my parents' basement, and I was recording my friends' bands, their friends' bands,
[and] then bands started coming from out of town, and it was just kind of the place to go and I
eventually realized, "Oh shit, I could make a job out of this."

In this business, if you provide a good experience, word of mouth is all the advertising you
really need, 'cause people in bands know people in bands. I finished recording an album, and
the drummer from the band hit me up to tell me about a space in a factory on the West Side
of Chicago that would be good for a studio. That's the place we're in now that we built about
eight years ago.

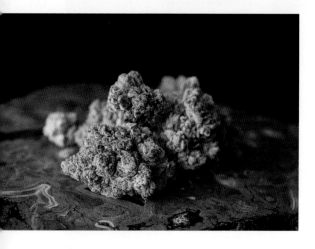

JW: Nice, and it looks like you're using all vintage recording equipment?

BG: Yeah, I love the way that it sounds, and it kind of forces you into a certain process that I think allows creativity to happen more frequently. With digital recording, a lot of times people say, "Oh, we'll fix that later," or "Let's just record it clean, and we'll figure it out later," but on tapes, you gotta make decisions. There are a lot of limitations, and you have to confront situations where you say, "OK, I can't do *this*, but how can I make it sound like I can?" It's a lot of messing around and trying to get the good tones. A lot of studios have tape machines and will work on tape, but there's only one other studio in town that's exclusively tape. We weren't really going for the niche thing. I was just being stubborn because I like working this way.

JW: When did cannabis come into your life?

BG: I started smoking pot in high school. I was dating a girl at the time who smoked cigarettes, and they just drove me nuts. So, after months of arguing about it, I landed on "If I smoke pot, will you quit smoking cigarettes?" and she agreed. We went to her friend's house and met the friend's boyfriend—this dude called "SoCal" because he was from Southern California. I definitely got the royal treatment. That first day, I smoked weed every single possible way there was to smoke weed. We started out with a blunt and then they were like, "This is how a bong works," then "This is how a steamroller works." Alright. "This is a spliff." Little did I know that meant there was tobacco in it, which is what I was against in the first place. I didn't think I was high. I was waiting to start tripping my balls off or something, and it just never really happened. Eventually, I just went on my way and skateboarded home, and then I got home, ate an entire pizza, and I thought, "Oh yeah, I'm definitely pretty high right now."

JW: Do you remember when you first realized it could have a creative effect on you?

BG: Leaving home and living with five other dudes, everyone's smoking pot all the time and just making music, so it just always went hand in hand. The thing I loved the most about getting stoned was that I always felt like no matter how many times I've heard a song, when I heard it

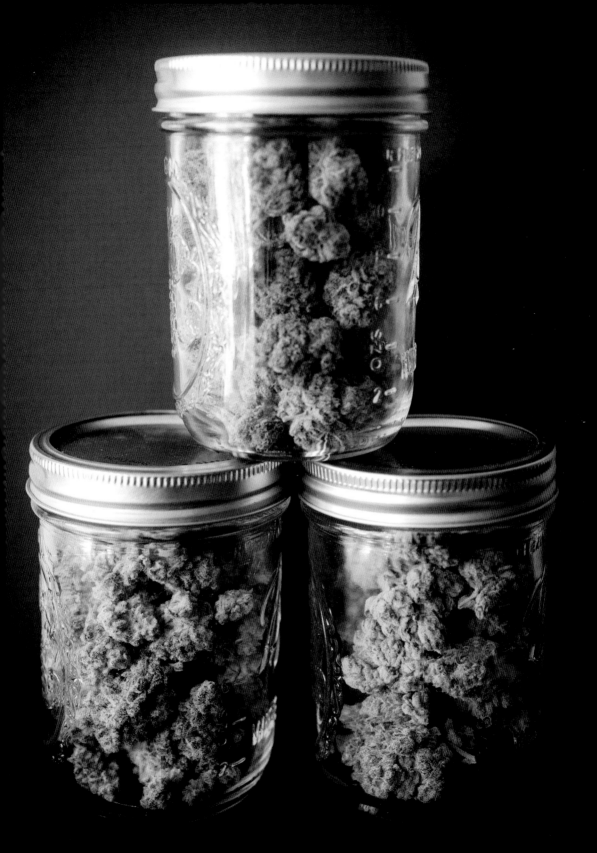

stoned it was like hearing it for the first time. I always thought that was a really valuable tool for making music because sometimes you get so wrapped up in it and you kinda lose total perspective; you don't even know what it sounds like anymore. You get stoned, and it changes your perspective. It's like you're hearing it how someone else would hear it. You're wiping your mind clean. It became a thing for me where I couldn't wait to smoke a little weed and listen to music. I was re-experiencing all of my favorite songs for the first time.

JW: So, what part does pot play in your creative process now?

BG: I like to be routine about things, especially with the recording process. I like to get the band set up, get everything dialed in, make sure everything's working and we're ready to get recording. Then, before we press record, you can smoke a little weed, and then the perspective comes.

JW: Does it help you get on the same page with musicians to smoke with them?

BG: There have definitely been numerous times where bands come in the studio, and they're a little uncomfortable. It's normally a very solid icebreaker. If they wanna smoke pot, that's when you start opening up and having more real conversations as opposed to just a business relationship. So, that bridges that gap a little, which is always nice. You're making music. It's art. You have to be comfortable when you do it.

JW: Are there any other ritualistic things you do to get in the creative headset?

BG: I normally like to get here an hour before the band shows up, get some coffee going, smoke some weed, just clean up the studio, make sure that we're ready for the day—anything that needs to be set up or anything that needs to be put away. Normally, if the timing is right, about 10 minutes before, I'll have a cigarette and then I'm ready to open the doors up, get ready for the band to come in.

JW: Wait, so you *are* smoking cigarettes after the whole point was to get your ex to quit?

BG: Hahaha. Yeah. That's a whole other story. It started with spliffs. A guy from a band I had in the studio was rolling something up and asked, "Do you want to go and take a hit of this? It's a spliff." And I'm like, "What does that mean? Is there tobacco in it? Oh, no, no, no, no." But we worked together for a few weeks, and at a certain point I realized I'm passing on a lot of free weed right now. So, I decided, fuck it, I'll try it. I took a nice big hit of it and then

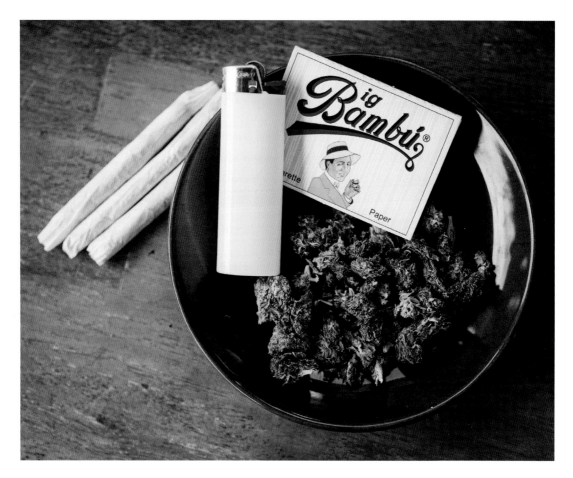

got immediately, insanely light-headed, spinning, I don't know what's gonna happen. Then 20 minutes later, I was like, "I kinda wanna do that again." That was it. I'm sold. I like smoking spliffs. Then one day I ran out of weed, went to a tobacco shop 'cause I wanted to smoke something, and I decided cigarettes aren't that bad.

JW: So that was legitimately pot acting as a gateway drug!

BG: Hahaha. One hundred percent. Yes. A gateway into smoking cigarettes, for sure.

JW: What does it feel like for you now? You just smoked a spliff and you're getting in the zone, can you describe what the sensations are?

BG: The word I always describe it as is "contrast." I feel like things start to separate. It almost feels like it starts with my stomach, moving up, and it's just washing away everything from before. I literally get stoned and forget what I was thinking about, and that's exactly what I wanted. To just start from scratch. Blank slate. And I think that's normally why I do it and what I achieve.

JW: Do you think of it as a mind expander or as an energy focuser or somewhere in between?

BG: I think it largely depends on what I'm doing. In a creative way, it's more mind-expanding. It's that classic thing of, "Oh, what if we get stoned and add this crazy backwards guitar?" That happens all the time, and then we're all sitting there like, "Wait…Should we…?" Then you listen to it the next day, and it was either a great idea or it's a terrible idea.

JW: Is the act of rolling the joint part of the ritual for you?

BG: Absolutely. It's almost down to a science. I've always wanted to take a video of me rolling a spliff 10 times and play the videos over each other. I bet it's almost exactly the same every time. I do half tobacco, half weed in the grinder, grind it up, and pour it out onto a record or something. Get it all together in a neat pile, then I'll get my paper out, get my crutch made, whether it's ripping a business card up or if I've got something else laying around, get the crutch rolled up, put it in, sprinkle the weed, roll it up, and smoke it.

JW: The filter? I've never heard it called a crutch before!

BG: Really? I learned it from that guy, SoCal!

JW: Do you still write music? How does cannabis play into that process?

BG: When I'm making music, I like to use it more, but I like to wait until I'm done for the day to get stoned. I like to be sober the whole time I write and record, and then when I hear it played back for the first time, I'm gonna hear it through a different perspective. I can judge it and see what it would sound like through someone else's ears.

JW: So, in that situation it becomes more of a tool for reflection than something for active creation?

BG: Yeah, and a lot of times it helps because at the end of a long day of fighting the fight, making the songs, I'll just be getting stoned, and be like, "Alright, I just hope this doesn't sound like shit." And then smoking gives you a little more confidence. You play it back, and you're like, "Oh yeah! It doesn't sound that bad!"

Kael Mendoza

chef

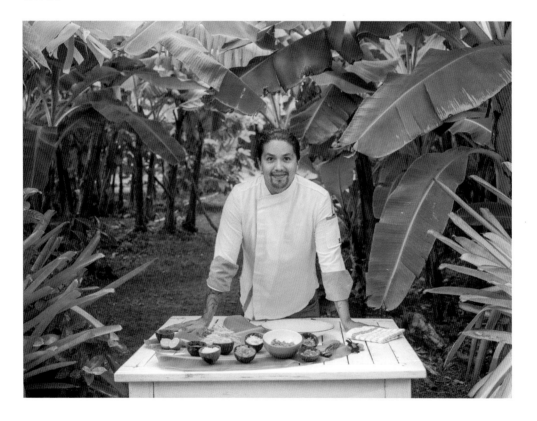

Some artists prefer to commit acts of creation while high. Sparking a joint before painting a mural or putting words to paper with a pipe nearby provides a heightened creative experience. For chef Kael Mendoza, cannabis's greatest benefit isn't what he can achieve in the kitchen while high, it's what happens outside of the kitchen. Mendoza most appreciates cannabis for the brainstorming sessions it inspires. For the ability to think of new and inventive ideas. For the first step in a larger process.

Back home, after a long day in the kitchen, he prepares for his smoke sessions with a pen and a notebook so he can record all the thoughts that come to him while his mind wanders

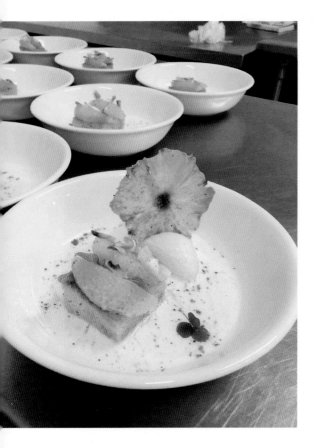

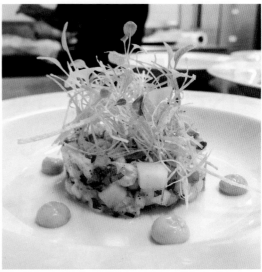

through imaginings of flavors, aromas, and new uses for common ingredients. Familiar recipes get a new spin. Anything from a song lyric to a popular flavor profile is broken down, analyzed, and incorporated into one of Mendoza's clever new creations.

Creativity isn't necessarily the goal for his smoke sessions, but it is a familiar and appreciated result. "I like to smoke," he begins, "It relaxes me, and then ideas can come up as my brain starts to make new connections." Through that relaxation and the mental space to explore, he often feels more capable of accessing the type of outside-the-box ideas that made him fall in love with the culinary arts.

Mendoza, who professionally goes by the moniker The Avocado Chef, hails from Mexico City but has studied food and culinary arts all over the world. After graduating from culinary school in Mexico in 2010, he traveled throughout the region of Catalonia in Spain to study with chefs at Michelin Star restaurants. Working with the chefs at El Racó de Can Fabes and El Celler de Can Roca introduced him to new concepts of what could be achieved with food through the lens of Catalan cuisine.

He spent the next few years exploring Caribbean flavors at a luxury resort in the Turks and Caicos, working in his third Michelin Star kitchen at Geranium in Copenhagen, Denmark, and learning large-scale food service as a banquet chef at a large hotel in Los Cabos, Mexico. With a diverse set of experiences under his belt, Mendoza was ready for an opportunity to focus in a small, boutique culinary environment. He accepted a position at Guana Island, where he worked for two years as a chef before being promoted to executive chef.

Guana Island embodies the classic, elegant yet simple, nature-filled environment you might picture when you think of an unspoiled Caribbean island. Located in the British Virgin Islands (BVI), the resort enjoys absolute privacy with no neighbors apart from the occasional iguana, tortoise, or flamingo visitor. As the chef responsible for feeding the resort's small collection of guests (there are only 18 rooms), Mendoza was free to experiment with ingredients, flavors, and techniques in ways that helped him grow as a culinary artist.

Because Guana Island maintains a private organic orchard, menus were often designed not according to the chef's whims, but around what was ripe and available that day. Spontaneous menus invented for specific ingredients allowed him to find more creativity and flexibility in his work. Common Caribbean flavors also provided ample inspiration.

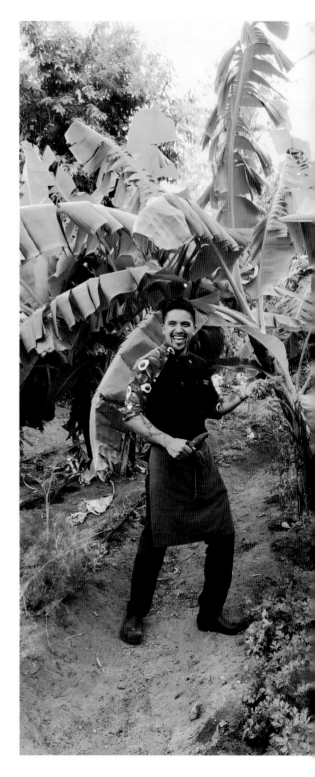

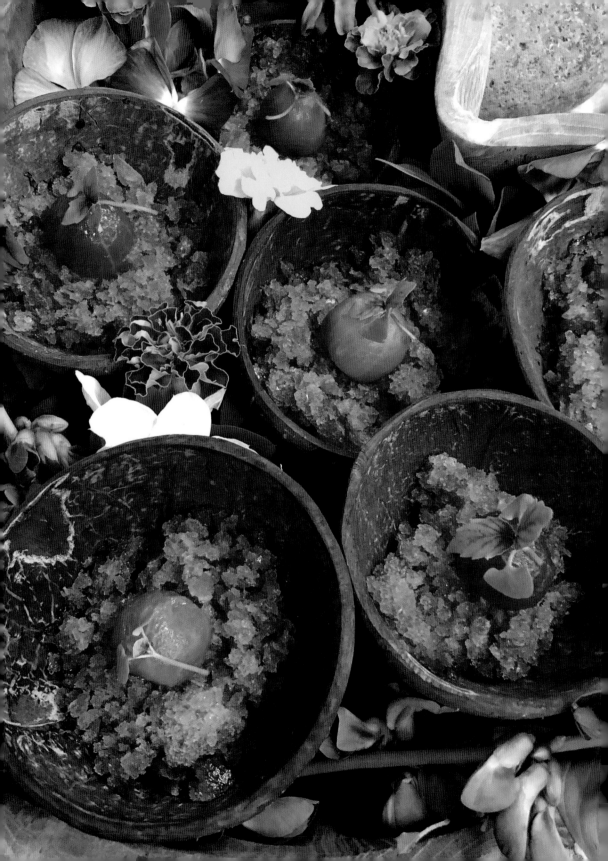

A day trip to Jost Van Dyke, a nearby island, resulted in one of Mendoza's favorite new creations, a take on the popular BVI cocktail: The Painkiller. "I was with a friend from the kitchen, and we were having some drinks and had a little bit to smoke. We were [lying] on the beach drinking Painkillers and I realized 'Wow, this is so tasty! It has all these flavors.' I realized we should make a dessert out of it. Take all of the ingredients and make something new. Why not?"

Mendoza soon perfected a dessert featuring all the flavors of the iconic Painkiller presented in a brand-new format: an orange cake with a coconut and rum foam served with pineapple sorbet, dried pineapple garnish, and fresh-ground nutmeg on top. He partially credits experiences like this with the expansive thinking he achieves after smoking, and partially with the invigoration he feels when he starts playing with ingredients.

"With weed, everything starts with ideas," he explains. "How is this going to taste served with that? Boom...And I just write ideas. The next day, once I'm starting to work in the kitchen and I have the products in my hand, I can really start to be creative."

In the kitchen, he always works with a clear mind. Cannabis puts him in too mellow of a state to want to be as active as his kitchen work requires, so he smokes to invent at night and arrives at work ready to experiment.

Inspiration and new skills or techniques are things Kael Mendoza seeks out anywhere he can: in cookbooks, in magazines, in smoke sessions with other chefs, and in the kitchens of masters. His continued desire to learn led him back home to Mexico, where he embarked on a two-year road trip in a Volkswagen van. The goal: to visit each of Mexico's states, experience the unique flavors and culinary traditions of each location, and offer his services in the kitchen in exchange for knowledge.

To culminate the experience, he plans to open a restaurant in Mexico that will celebrate all he has learned about the country's diverse cultures and foods. When the time comes to create menus and design his own endeavor, Mendoza's brainstorming sessions will benefit not only from cannabis but from the exciting collection of ideas he's gathered over the course of two years as he pushes himself to reinvent old favorites and explore the most delicious flavors of Mexico.

Mark Karan

musician

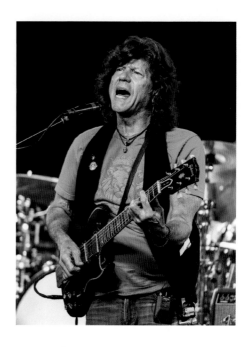

Mark Karan has had a long and storied career as a guitarist and singer. Best known as the lead guitarist of the band RatDog, with a post-Grateful Dead Bob Weir, Karan has also performed with a number of top acts in the world of blues, rock, reggae, funk, and Americana.

JW: Can you give me a bit of background on your artistic journey?

MARK KARAN: Well, I'm a musician, singer, songwriter, guitar player, producer, and I was the lead guitar player in RatDog. I have always done music as my profession and also as my passion. I had the joyful experience of being able to participate in the Haight–Ashbury and all of that stuff. So I got introduced to pot pretty early. I first discovered pot when I was about 11 years old, and I first discovered LSD when I was about 13.

I have a history of some addiction. I've been sober from booze and cocaine for about 36 years, and about 16 years into that sobriety, I decided that pot had never been my difficulty. I had 16 years away from the booze and the blow, and I didn't really feel heavily at risk or anything, so I started doing what a lot of people sort of lovingly, jokingly call "the Marijuana Maintenance program." It was my version of sobriety. I would still be sober from all the hard drugs and the booze and whatnot, but to me, pot and psychedelics never fit into those categories, and I think of them as having a lot of benefits that those other kinds of drugs don't offer. And that served me for about 20 years.

JW: Did you have any transition from enjoying cannabis just for the social aspects and the joy of being high, toward, "Oh, I can use this productively. This can help me tap into my creativity?"

MK: I don't know that those two things were ever separate. I think they developed simultaneously, and in some ways are almost the same thing. I've always thought of pot as assisting my creativity. The reason that I *have* puffed pretty regularly when playing has been, to some degree, medicinal, but it's also been social. That's all mixed up in the same stuff, because what I do a lot of the time is out in public. I do have a background with recording, and certainly pot can be very helpful in the creativity involved in that process, but the majority of what I've done has been live music. It's kind of a combination of the social thing and the creative, especially since I started playing with some of the guys from The Grateful Dead back in '98. That type of music requires a pretty open mind and a lot of creative, explorational spirit, because so much of it is improvisational as opposed to something that's written and rehearsed. I wouldn't wanna do an improvisationally based gig without puffing.

JW: What effect does smoking have on your creativity?

MK: In my experience, puffing makes my editor shut the hell up. I can fall into that trap of feeling judged by my fellow musicians or feeling judged by the audience or feeling like I suck. And even though you *know* it's not true, those little noises in your head can have a lot of power. With pot, I find that I'm able to follow the trail into the music. I get so deeply involved in the music, I'm probably not a very satisfying performer in terms of smiling and looking up and being interactive and all of that kind of performer stuff, but I think I'm probably a very rewarding performer from the perspective of people that really love seeing creativity in action, because that's what happens.

JW: So you feel like it's enhancing rather than dampening the creative experience?

MK: Oh, absolutely, yeah. The way I envision it inside my head, my ears get very big, and I can hear everything that everybody's doing. All of it comes with its own set of inspired ideas and responses. For me, that's the big difference between a drug like blow, booze, speed— those kinds of drugs. To me, they're all designed to shut you down. It's like, "I'm in pain. I don't wanna feel anymore. Let me use this drug." I look at them as drugs that are designed to make you vacate. Pot and psychedelics both are designed to open your mind and open your heart.

JW: How does smoking pot affect the physical dexterity part of what you do?

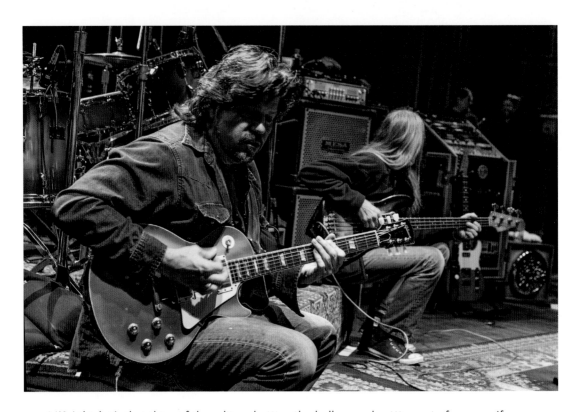

MK: I think it's that thing of the editor shutting the hell up and getting out of my way. If I'm feeling self-conscious, my brain leads me to go do stuff that I already know how to do, which is boring. When I get like that, I get more self-conscious, especially if I notice that I'm trapped in that loop. Then, yeah, my actual physical movements can get impeded; they can get clunky. That's what happens when I'm not puffing. When I am puffing, it's not a direct connection to my physicality, but it's my mental process and spiritual and emotional process. I'm plugging into the flow such that my body seems to follow suit. Movements become more automatic and easy. It's the mental processes that can get in the way of our physicality or physical flow. Pot quiets a lot of that down so that what would naturally happen is allowed to happen.

JW: Have you noticed any difference in the type of energy you get based on variety or strain?

MK: Absolutely, yeah. For creativity, I absolutely prefer sativa. I find that the indicas are great, and I love the flavors and the smells and the look. That's a big piece of how I relate to pot smoking too. Some people look at alcohol like it's a means to get drunk, and so box wine is just fine. Of course, that's part of it. I wanna get high, but I wanna get high with a

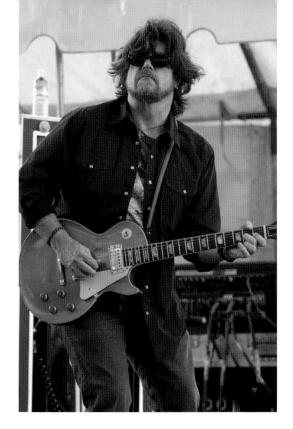

classy, high-end experience. I wanna take it out of a nice jar. I wanna feel a squishy bud, and smell it, and look at the beautiful crystals, and break it up carefully, and roll a good joint that's nice and even burning, and appreciate the taste. It's a whole experience. As far as effects, sativa seems to be more psychedelic, which is what gets my creative font flowing more.

JW: Do you smoke when you intend to be creative, or do you smoke and creativity is a byproduct?

MK: Well, I've found myself at a strange turning point right now where I'm actually examining whether or not I wanna keep puffing. I have become habituated in ways that I don't find constructive. I don't want to feel that I'm checking out or like pot has become—I hate to use the dreaded word—a version of an addiction or an unhealthy self-medication. It's really tough, though, because I still play music, and when I play music, I still wanna get high to enhance that experience. So I don't really relish the idea of stopping puffing, but I'm feeling kind of a pretty potent need to stop some of the behavior that I've been doing just so I can get more in touch with myself.

JW: Do you think you could achieve the same creative energy via other pathways? Is it the act of undergoing a sort of state change with pot that inspires creativity, or is it something else?

MK: I don't believe that it's just a state change that makes creativity happen—not just any kind of state change. It's gotta be a more specific kind of change. When I puff, it feels like my neural pathways in my brain expand. I get access to pathways that don't normally seem to be there. I've always had a belief that I should be able to recreate those pathways via some sort of meditative or spiritual practice, like getting to some version of consciousness or connectedness, and I do meditate, but I haven't really noticed that it enhances my creativity. I want it to! I love the idea of it, but thus far it hasn't been my experience.

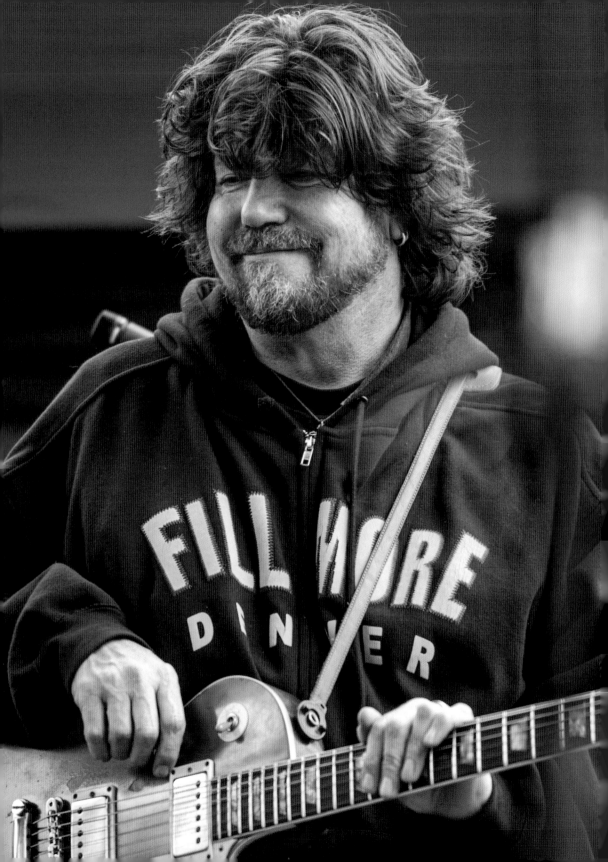

JW: Is there a perfect threshold of how high you want to be for achieving creativity?

MK: For me, a couple of hits is enough to do what I'm talking about. I don't need to be hella stoned; I just need to have become a little altered. If it's good pot, two, maybe three hits, and I'm ready to play music, and that will usually get me through a whole set.

JW: Does music gel better if you've smoked with the group that you're performing with?

MK: If you're gonna be doing something in the group setting like playing music, it's cool to connect before you hit the stage. But that can just be catching up. It doesn't seem to make much difference to me if we all puff together, or if everyone puffs separately, or if one or two of the people don't puff it all. That's one of the things that I used to believe: that everybody needed to be on the same page. I don't believe that anymore. I have enough friends, a couple of whom historically were heavy pot consumers, that decided not to consume anymore at all, but they're still very involved in improvisational, Grateful Dead-rooted music. They still seemed to be really happy with their levels of creativity, and I've been really happy with what they've come up with musically, so now I no longer believe that everybody needs to be stoned or on the same page. It's me. I need to have access.

JW: Is performing with others the most creatively fulfilling for you?

MK: One of the things that happens in a group setting when I'm playing music, it's a little strange, but I tend to experience some version of what I would call telepathy. It's something I experienced even more intensely when close friends and I would drop large quantities of acid together. We could read each other without speaking. That happens in music with weed. If I'm high, and my head is down and I have soft focus, I'm not looking at anything or really thinking about anything. I'm not thinking about playing music. I'm not planning what I'm gonna play next or examining what I just played or tripping on the fact that I just made a mistake—it's none of that. I just let go. Shut up and see what happens. And when I'm in that space of trusting the creative muse, I kind of hear other people's ideas, and they spark ideas for me and open up pathways—places to go. So that's what I'm looking for when I'm puffing. Can I open up these lines of communication?

Playing guitar by myself, I can get real creative, but the super, super joy comes in the creativity that happens when the whole is greater than the sum of the parts. The group thing; it's a real joy. It's a real release for me.

Colton Clifford

photographer, visual artist, and performer

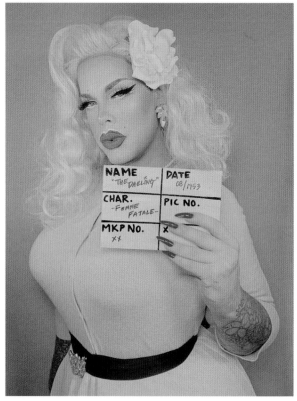

Clifford as The Darling

In many circumstances, photography is the ultimate truth-teller's tool. It's a means of documenting life with little room for interpretation. If the camera captures it, it was there, as depicted. But photography also presents opportunities for creating illusions and fantasies, building environments and worlds, and telling stories that repackage reality into something else entirely. Those fantastical and illusory aspects of photography were the elements that first drew Colton Clifford to find their artistic passion. For them, it's less about documenting what's there on the surface, and more about expanding reality into a realm of fantastical wonder.

Clifford creates rich, cinematic, and often ethereal portraits and self-portraits of performers in drag. Sometimes they're posed like pouty pinups in a pop-art explosion of color, tinsel, and light. Sometimes they're represented with a classic, noir, old-Hollywood feel. But in every photo, Clifford's primary focus is to showcase the model how they see themselves and want to be seen.

"When I photograph," they explain, "the idea is to take queer existence, put it in heteronormative landscapes, and allow the constructs of each of those elements to challenge each other. There's a lot of set decorating, a lot of lighting and posing, and it all helps to create this kind of magical illusion."

Now, in their adopted hometown of New Orleans, Clifford has fully embraced their place in the drag community through photography, digitally drawn portraits of drag performers, and, most recently, through live performance. The Darling, Clifford's drag persona, has expanded beyond the still-image and onto the stage, something which has provided a valued creative outlet.

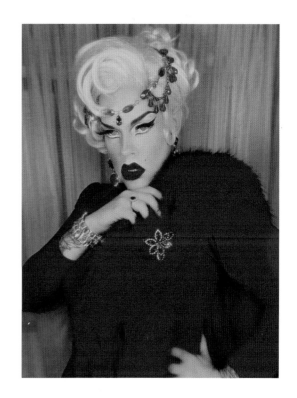

"Photography was the thing that truly gave me a space to let this energy out. It was a kind of mental release on its own, but I felt like my photographs might have a different impact if I knew what it was like to perform on stage. I started drag as a research idea, but then this world exploded where every expression of self is celebrated and looked at as beautiful, whether you're plus size, or thin, or brown, or white, or femme-presenting, or masc-presenting, a queen, a king, nonbinary…Now, artistically and creatively, I'm more liberated by performing than I am by photographing."

Clifford's explorations of art, both visual and performance-based, have always engaged with the idea of breaking down barriers. It's a pursuit that also connects to their appreciation of cannabis. "When I smoke, it's more for a creative purpose than it is for relaxing," they tell me. "I find myself able to bring down walls that block me from

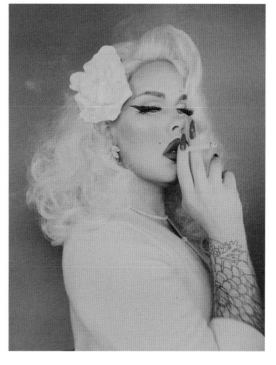

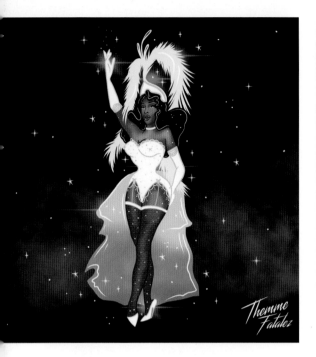

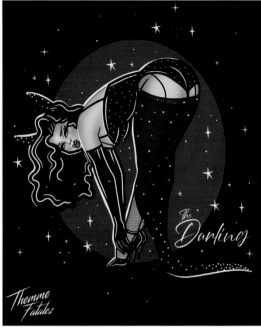

creating. Whether it's drag or painting or photography, those walls stop me from exploring. With drag, you're giving so much of yourself to an audience. Anxiety flares up, but if I smoke, I can function and enjoy the things I'm doing. It allows me to be comfortable in my actions as a person and be more confident in them. I'm more willing to take creative risks."

A lot goes into preparing for a drag performance. As Clifford tells it, there's not only the physical aspect of getting into character, with costumes, hair, glue, makeup, and a fair amount of shaving, there's also the mental aspect of getting ready to engage with the audience. For the uninitiated, the sorts of burlesque drag shows that Clifford performs in are extremely interactive. The audience cheers, shouts, flirts, dances, and sometimes tries to climb on stage (usually rowdy bachelorette parties). Performers are in the thick of it, so there's not much room for hesitation or anxiety. Add to that the fact that most audiences are either drunk or high, or drunk *and* high, and smoking pot before a show becomes a necessary means of getting on the same page as your audience.

Clifford understands that audiences come to their shows to escape and enjoy the fantasy. "Smoking or eating an edible in that situation allows me to be on the same page with them so we can access this euphoric area together. This world exists because everybody comes to feel their most beautiful and express themselves in an honest and vulnerable way. It's this

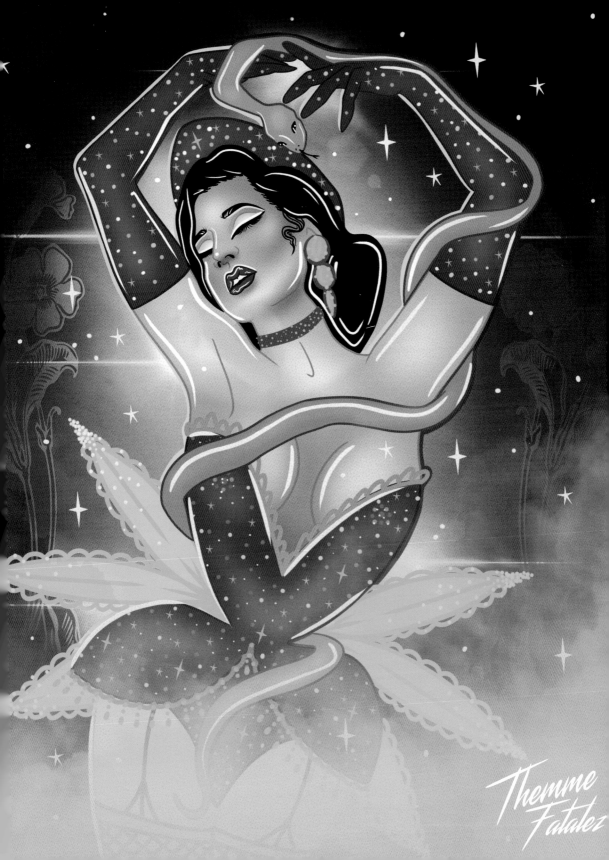

Themme
Fatalez

very celebratory space. We're celebrating the audience as much as they're celebrating us, so it's an equalized balance."

In photography and digital illustration, cannabis also provides them a path through nagging voices of self-doubt, but timing is everything. For visual arts, the first smoke of the day is usually the most potent and provides the greatest flow state and rush of ideas. In their high state, imaginative leaps feel more accessible, so visual fantasy is easier to believe in and create. "When I'm smoking creatively, I want that feel, that rush of escapism. I'm dissociating from the parts of me that want to over-edit or control my existence." Whether it's in photographs or illustrations, or on stage as The Darling, Colton Clifford is a master of the multidisciplinary and a weaver of fantasy.

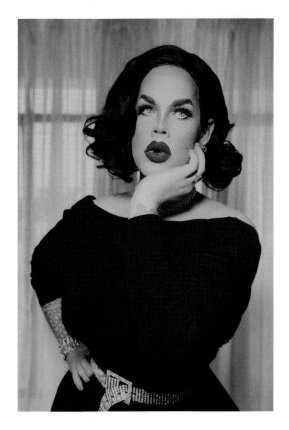

Even in our day-to-day existence, Clifford believes we could all use a little more fantasy, self-love, and self-expression in our lives. "There are mornings where I wake up, look in the mirror, and think 'No, absolutely not. I do not care for this.' It's really easy as a human to get sucked in by that toxic feeling and believe it. But the second I smoke, even just one hit, I love myself and I'm confident in myself. I worked hard to create this version of me, to care about the people around me, and to love them in the same way that I love myself. Cannabis taught me how to love others and see others' beauty. We're all learning a bit more love of others and self-love right now. I think if everybody smoked a little bit, then they might see how dumb and superficial it is that we're so hard on ourselves and each other."

Robert Poehler
theatre director and professor

Robert Poehler (not his real name) is a college professor in a prestigious theatre program. He holds a Ph.D. in theatre and has been focused on theatrical processes for well over a decade. While he spends most of his professional time teaching, he directs plays and advises students in their own theatrical productions as well.

JW: Can you give me a bit of background on your artistic journey?

ROBERT POEHLER: I really got interested in making theatre as a high school student. It was about the formation of community, and maybe there was some vague idea about self-expression. In college I was excited by the immediate appeal of spending my days in a studio with other people, trying to arrive at collective thought and expression. After college I was going to pursue the dream of being an independent theatre director, and did for a little bit, but in America, the dream of middle-class stability reigns supreme, and so I went to graduate school. Since then, I've been working in a university context most of the time and it's nice because it's a sheltered space in which resources are plentiful and time is allocated to creative activity. In the company of people that I consider artists, I probably would not call myself an artist unless I get to qualify it as a "teaching artist" or an "artist scholar," because most of my energy isn't put toward making art. Instead, I teach in a discipline that is about art-making, and part of my responsibility is to make art for and with the undergraduates that I teach.

JW: Do you believe that cannabis makes you more creative?

RP: I've been wrestling with how I'm going to describe this because at one end of the spectrum, there's a fantasy about artists who arrive at inspiration through substances, and I don't want to say that that's not the truth. In fact, I'm really taken with intentional applications of psychedelics, of marijuana, of all forms of substances. In my experience, I haven't sat down and said, "OK, it's time to be creative. Let's get high." Marijuana is basically a daily activity for me, and mostly I think of it as a way of reducing stress. Sometimes getting high means I don't have to care so much, and in some ways, that release from the pressures of caring, of expectation, of logical measurement of productivity, of priorities that the rational mind sets for itself, the release from that can open gateways to creative thinking. I guess I also don't locate the entire creative process in a period of being high. It's the gateway. It's an opening.

JW: What happens once you open that gateway?

RP: I find myself entering this state of release and discovering kind of accidentally that it has freed thought patterns that have been constrained throughout the day in the rehearsal room. When I'm lucky, it might lead me, especially in the early stages of a project, to a thing that I have called a kind of "spirit flight," a lush visual and aural imagining that strikes an inner resonance. It's that inner resonance that I'm always looking for as an artist.

I think our bodies are our best critics, so I'll ask my students, "How do you know when something's interesting?" For me, it's a bodily experience, and I find that marijuana attunes me to that kind of response in myself. It allows me to trust intuition and to follow thoughts further than I might in a sober state. I don't use it instrumentally; I sort of arrive at creative moments through it accidentally. Every once in a while, you buy a bag that does something different and that brings you closer to a productive creative state of mind.

JW: How do you incorporate that state of mind into the larger creative process?

RP: The sort of spirit flight that I might achieve on a really great high becomes an experience that I have to sleep on so I can filter it and remember it and figure out how to apply it subconsciously, and it's there in the background as a memory and as a guiding principle, but it becomes the basis for the creative process, not the creative process itself.

JW: So it's more like a philosophical pathway that sets you up for the creative process later?

RP: Yeah, and I think the beautiful thing is that it often feels unconstrained by expectations. Some people might want to call it "inspiration" because it seems to strike out of the blue. Other people might think "I can make this happen by getting high right now," but in my experience, I can't *make* it happen, but it might be more likely to happen if I can relax a part of my mind that constrains creativity. That's the metaphor I like: my mind constrains creativity and marijuana relaxes the constraints.

JW: I like that too. Has cannabis always had this elevating effect on your thought process?

RP: Hanging out with the theatre crowd in college, pot was the primary engine of socialization, so my introduction to habitual smoking was about being with others and sharing experiences. Those experiences, especially in the young stoner mind, are often creative. I remember being with people and literally imagining other worlds that we felt we could inhabit in our state. I think in some ways it was both a curative to the pressured environment of academia for an 18-year-old, and a way of socializing. It was an exciting alternate state of mind.

JW: You were saying earlier that smoking and creativity isn't a causative *A* results in *B* kind of thing for you. I wonder if people who value creativity in their lives just tend to gravitate toward a state of altered consciousness. It's not as much a direct pathway of "I smoke, and I'm now more creative." Maybe it's more of a Venn diagram: "I am a person who smokes. I enjoy that unconstrained aspect of my mind. I am also a person who creates."

RP: I think the idea that it's related to a state of mind that already exists is important. Anybody can smoke, but certain people are drawn to it and make habits of it. Some people hate the loss of control. For me, the loss of control is freeing.

I like that what you're saying implies creativity isn't something that can be imported through the use of a substance. It has to be something that already exists in your thought patterns, behaviors, ways of presenting yourself—and marijuana can be a catalyst or an aid to allowing that to come forward. I totally believe that people who want to spend their lives in creative environments may become more and more comfortable with living inside another brain state. It offers an escape from the pressures of constantly operating in a space governed by productivity, rationality, and logic.

JW: Some artists say it's more expansive in terms of the types of thoughts they can have while high. Others say that pot gives them more of a focusing-down kind of energy. For many, it's both. What is it for you?

RP: I think it's both expansion and focus. There's an expansion of possibility and also the ability to dive deep into a thing you've discovered in your expansive state.

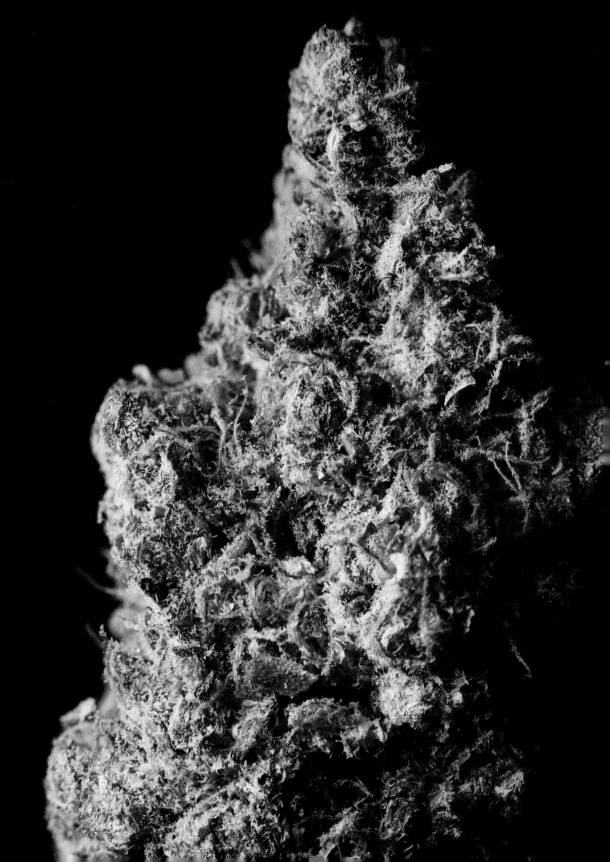

JW: I think it also comes back to what you were saying earlier about needing time to process and think about your new creative leaps. It's probably a good idea if you write stoned and edit sober.

RP: Absolutely. Because if you're not employing this kind of multistage editing, you're just getting high and making something for other stoners. The logic will only be there for the stoned mind.

JW: I think in some applications that might be enough, like in visual arts, painting, or collage. But in terms of writing or other pursuits where you're asking people to join you on some kind of linear journey that they need to comprehend in any state of mind, you need that second revision.

RP: In writing, your reader needs to comprehend according to an established network of meaning that they already understand: syntax, structure, theory.... You can't just suspend that. But in some ways, every painting has to teach you how to read it anyway.

JW: So in practical application, what does your creative process look like? Where does cannabis come in?

RP: The foundation of my creative process is built on lots of prep, analysis, decision-making, and rehearsal. After weeks or months of work, I'm looking for the moment when my brain is able to collect all of the structures, architectures, and meaning in a play and make something even more meaningful out of it through image and action. Most often, that happens after a rehearsal. I get high, and it feels like the jumble of questions that I left the rehearsal room with settle like shells floating downward through the ocean. As they lie still on the floor, something else moves and, preconsciously, the elements start to reform themselves in patterns, and I start to internally see things that resonate. I allow a new logic of causality to move the image forward and to pull other things I've been thinking about into it and make sense of them. If it's going well, I get a tingle up my spine, and that's my signal to not think and just let the daydream continue, because it's my rational mind or my body saying, "Oh, this is good, let's not ask why yet."

JW: So it seems like that post-rehearsal solo-reflection is a key part of the process.

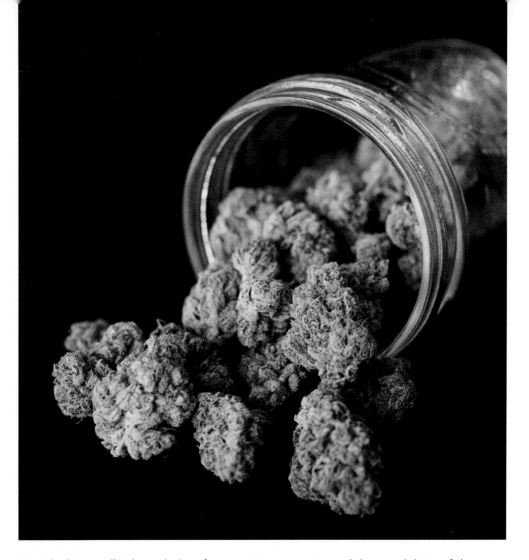

RP: I think I actually channel a lot of my creative energy toward the possibilities of the decompression moments of being high after the work. Because the things that I think are important about preparing for a directing process are actually about limiting external influences instead of expanding them. For example, as soon as I know I'm going to direct a play, I will not watch anyone else's version of it. I will not look at images of it. I want to create a space of thought and feeling that is separate from outside influences. I want to protect the possibilities of my stoned engagement with that material as the sort of imagistic source that I'll use. I also think many of the other activities of preparation are sort of banal and boring. They're rooted in methods of intellectual labor. Maybe that's why it's so important to have high time.

JW: So the high time is acting as your reward for building the foundation and achieving the other aspects of the process?

RP: I think that's fair, but it's not just a reward separate from the process. I've done the work and now I'm at a point where I can let my brain relax enough to let it play.

JW: You talked a bit about your early experiences of being high and how that was a largely communal experience. I know making theatre is very communal as an art, but do you ever introduce the cannabis aspect into your collaborations?

RP: Well, because I'm in academics, it's not a great idea to get all the students high, but when I'm working with other professional collaborators—especially designers or choreographers—then the best thing that can happen after working really hard all day at rehearsal is going to get stoned together. I think in that situation, marijuana becomes a lubricant to getting on the same page. We're both open to suggestion in ways that our minds might normally shut out. We can have one of those late-night stoner talks where your dialogue creates the world that you're both living in, and you can find solutions to problems that are collaboratively built if we can enter a similar brain state together.

JW: So now that sounds more like a reversal of the process. Write sober, edit stoned.

RP: Totally. I have been talking about this as if there's a single example where I do work and get high and then there's a product, but the truth is that a rehearsal process takes place over months or a year. So, there is a cycle, a constant back and forth. All day, I'm sober and I'm working, and at night I process and expand upon, or focus on, or check for resonance, or solve problems. Then I sleep and, in the morning, those things get translated back into rational behavior, and I go apply them, and then I discover new things that night.

JW: What happens to your process if you don't have access to cannabis?

RP: Well, last week I ran out and I found that creative thought erupts elsewhere. I had very vivid dreams that were incredibly realistic but also had the flavor of an inaccessible logic of meaning. They felt very much like an art piece. I feel like I can actually have an experience of stoner thought without being stoned, and that's maybe just because my brain is so used to that state and way of thinking that I'm not sure I absolutely need the chemical to go there anymore.

Mark McDowell

multidisciplinary artist

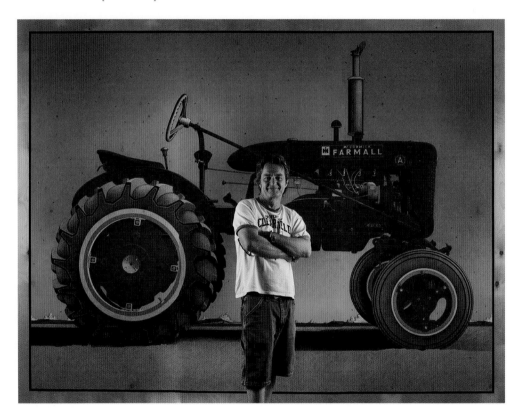

Mark McDowell sees art as a way of life. Artists, he explains, "need to do a lot of things. If you're an artist, the biggest window that you can give yourself with your skill sets is the greatest pathway to success. For many artists, the greatest success is to be able to make a living doing what you want to do. For me personally, being an artist is a whole lot more about working with my mind, and my wits, and my skill sets, mostly to avoid having a regular job."

McDowell certainly is an artist with a wild collection of skill sets. He's been a circus performer. He's a musician in a band. He owns and operates a publishing house through

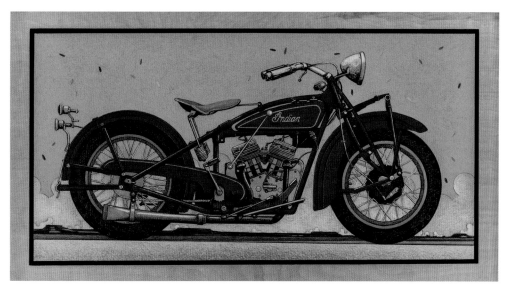

1928 Indian Scout

which he helps artists realize book projects and portfolio collections. He designs. He consults on projects great and small. He advises up-and-coming artists, and he collaborates in just about any medium. Each of those skill sets has led him to a life filled with art, and, as he happily tells me, it has successfully kept him from having to fall back on a brief post-college career of hot-tar roofing in the desert.

Living and working as a founding member of the Cattle Track Arts Compound, an artist colony in Scottsdale, AZ, McDowell spends his time floating mentally and physically through a constantly rotating collection of projects. On the morning we spoke, he had already participated in two design consulting meetings and had a full afternoon of other project work to handle before he could go into the studio to complete a drawing he'd been working on for a few weeks. Working this way fulfills his desire to help budding artists achieve their goals, just as someone once helped him on his journey. It fulfills his desire to keep busy and engaged in the arts, and it fulfills his desire to avoid hot tar at all costs.

These days, his personal artistic pursuit comes in the form of bold, colorful illustrations of various sizes and scopes. He draws subjects from landscapes to classic farm machinery using colored pencils and birchwood panels. It's very deliberate and time-consuming work. A single large-scale drawing of a tractor took him two years to create, but he loves doing it.

Central to McDowell's focus for all the projects he engages is the philosophy that art only happens by doing. "A lot of people say they're artists and then end up at Starbucks talking

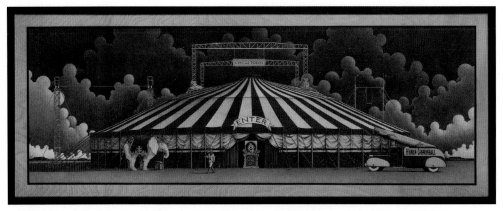

Circus Today

about it all the time. My cofounder of the arts compound, who was born here 80 years ago, says, 'No lazy sons of bitches.' I like to temper that a little bit. I tell people, 'Look, if you just wanna talk about it, go up to Starbucks. That's where everybody is at. If you wanna put your gloves on and do it, then let's do it.'"

When it comes to physically making art, navigating the creative process, and engaging completely with the tasks at hand, McDowell is a definite proponent of cannabis. He started smoking pot in the 1970s. As a young pot smoker, it began as a social thing centralized around music and concerts and geeking out about the Rolling Stones' impressive light show. In his adulthood, smoking pot isn't about intoxication. It represents a way of getting his thoughts in order, preparing for the day, and jump-starting creative pursuits.

"My work is not dependent on me catching a buzz. I see myself a little bit like a juggler. I've got a lot of projects going, and I want to be able to carry them through with aplomb. I want to make it appear effortless. Much of what I smoke pot for is to slow down my thinking a little bit. There's a lot going on, and if all you're doing is thinking, you're not doing. Sometimes smoking a little pot in the morning—you know, have a cup of coffee, have my breakfast, do my exercises, smoke a little pot—I can start to focus."

Over the years, other artists have expressed to him that they can't start to paint until all their brushes are clean, or that the best art is made when your house is in order—laundry folded, dishes done, bills paid. For McDowell, smoking pot helps get his house in order. It clarifies the intention and eliminates distracting thoughts that could divert him from his projects. He doesn't believe that pot makes him more creative, but that isn't to say that it doesn't help him in his creative work.

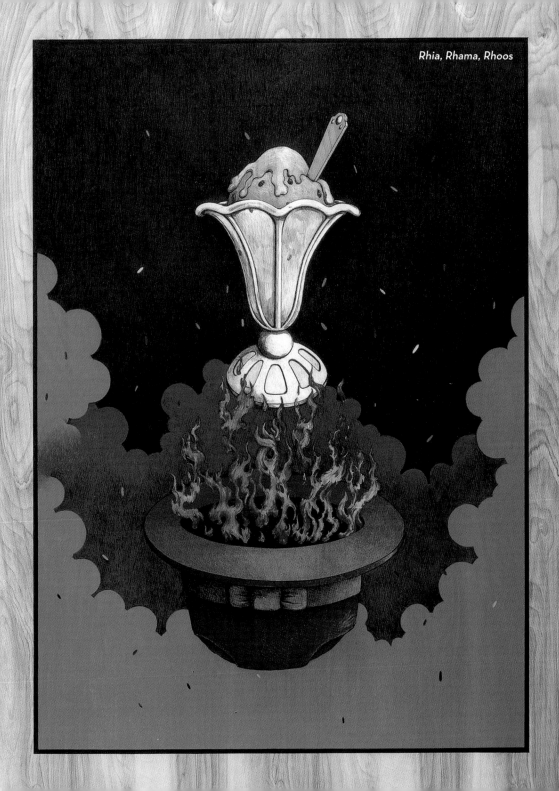

Rhia, Rhama, Rhoos

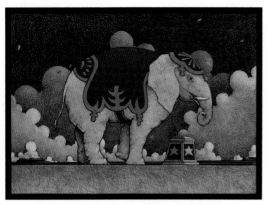

Circus Elephant

He explains, "Some people would say, 'Yeah, it makes me more creative,' but I would challenge that. I would say that their thinking process day-to-day-to-day is shielding or obfuscating their creative nature. You look at kids with a pile of wooden blocks on the floor making stuff—that's creative expression. They're not smoking any weed to get there, but then as they get in school, they gotta do homework, and they gotta do chores. Later, they gotta pay taxes and make a living and raise the kids. It clutters that childlike quality. We live in an information-rich society where people have a whole lot of shit to think about, and so I would maintain that smoking a joint steps you back a little bit from all the shit you have to think about."

After 50 years of smoking pot, a mild sativa offers his ideal sort of high, but he's not hitting the dispensaries looking at THC percentages or chasing appealing strain names. Like most other aspects of his life, he keeps it simple. He grows his weed in the same garden where he cultivates tomatoes, chili peppers, and basil. "I don't particularly need anything that's gonna make me see Jesus or make me wanna get on the couch with a bag of Oreos and a Three Stooges movie. That's unproductive to me. I smoke it in my workday."

In McDowell's experience, the first 15 minutes of any project are the hardest. That's when the day-to-day minutiae can invade your thoughts and overwhelm the first few embers of creativity just when they need to be stoked. If you can get through the first 15 minutes, you're engrossed. You're on a roll. For him, smoking a joint is the path to engaging in those first 15 minutes. Whether it's a consulting project, a drawing, or laying out a new portfolio, after the first 15 minutes, he's locked in, and the rest tends to flow on its own. The key is to silence distractions by any means necessary.

"I'm old," he tells me. "At this point, I've mastered what works. If something in your life is bothering you, get rid of it. If something in your life needs to be fixed, get on it because if you're a creative, you're only gonna be happy if you're following the muse and if it's giving you something back."

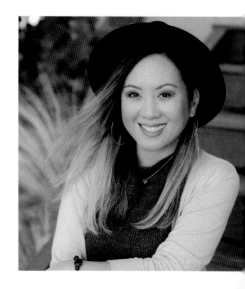

ARTIST INTERVIEW

Kay Villamin
entrepreneur and photographer

Kay Villamin is the cofounder and CEO of Hush Chicago, a full-service events and marketing agency for the cannabis industry. Hush Chicago focuses particularly on minority-owned businesses and startups who are also social equity applicants. Making an equal and diverse marketplace in the cannabis industry is one of their top priorities in business. Prior to founding Hush Chicago, Villamin worked professionally as a full-service photographer for much of her career.

JW: Can you tell me about yourself and what your artistic journey has been?

KAY VILLAMIN: I've lived in Chicago since 1993. Prior to that, I was living in the Philippines. Ever since I was a child, I've enjoyed creative things. I was always drawing; I was always painting. My mom was raising us by herself while my dad was here petitioning for us to come over to America, but even though she wasn't working, she left a lot to do the shopping, and she would leave me with a babysitter or a relative. I hated when she would leave, but one of the things that kept me company was making art. I had an active imagination.

Later, I was lucky enough to go to a high school that allowed you to choose a major, so I chose to do art. In my third year, my school opened a darkroom, and that's when photography started for me. I was only 17, and it was my first experience using a film camera, developing my own film, developing my own photos, spending hours at a time in the darkroom, and that's when I realized: I love this. This is home. I attribute a lot of the profound and really creative moments I had in the darkroom to the fact that I was using cannabis. That was the time when I felt like myself and I felt most at home, like "This is where I'm supposed to be." After that, I chose to go to Columbia College and pursue photography. So I did that and explored a lot of different types of photography.

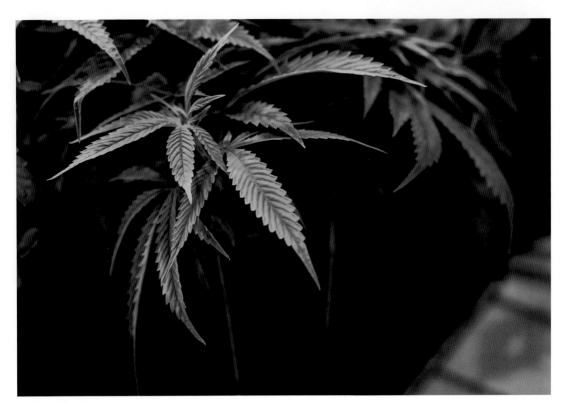

JW: You've worked as a professional photographer for most of your career?

KV: After I graduated, I worked in a photography studio in Evanston, where I stayed for eight years. That's where I was exposed to all kinds of professional photography that I didn't learn in school. I went on to start a photography studio with another photographer I met there. We decided we could do it on our own, so we made a plan, we saved up all the money to buy our own equipment, and we quit our jobs. We ran that business successfully for about six years, but then after a while, I realized it wasn't fulfilling for me anymore. Ever since I left school and started doing photography for work, I didn't pick up the camera just for me anymore—just to create. It was always for someone else.

Then, in early 2017, my dad got sick. He's better now, but at the time it really shook my world. That's when I decided it was time to stop everything that didn't serve me. It was time for me to stop and look around and decide what my purpose was. That's how things evolved and eventually got me to where I am in the cannabis industry.

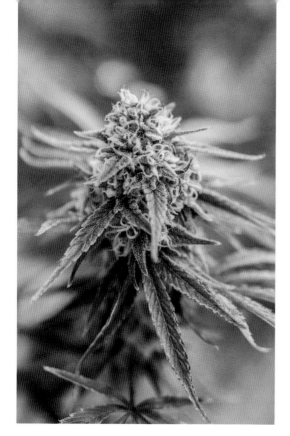

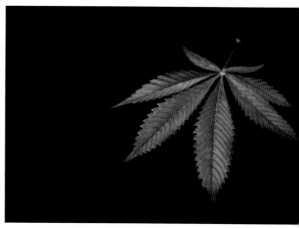

JW: OK, so let's backtrack. When did cannabis come into your life?

KV: It's been with me for about 18 years. It's like my longest relationship!

JW: Do you believe it makes you more creative?

KV: Oh yeah! Yeah, absolutely. A lot of my profound moments, my best ideas, answers to a lot of my questions, happen with cannabis. Just seeing things at literally that higher level, it gives you perspective, which then makes you more creative and be more open to different things. I feel like it activates parts of your brain, wakes up certain receptors that weren't awake. It helps you explore the things around you more and those things have a different meaning when you're up there—when you're high.

JW: Do you remember when you first realized it was affecting your creativity?

KV: I remember the precise moment, actually. I was in the darkroom, putting my print through the fixer, about to wash it. I was just swirling the image around, and I thought, "Oh my God, *this* is creation. *This* is art. This is something I literally captured in that moment, and I'm bringing it back to life and preserving it." I remember that moment in the darkroom and that was when I decided, this is what I'm gonna do for the rest of my life—or at least a huge chunk of my life.

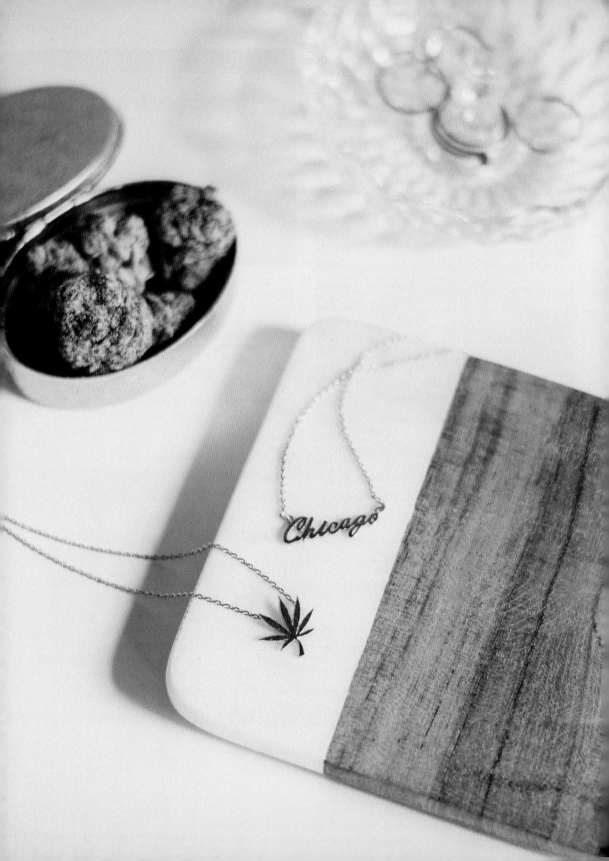

Around that time, I also first discovered the very spiritual effects of cannabis through music. Music has always been a very big part of my life, and so listening to music high for the first time, I realized I was hearing different things. Hearing different levels. I felt like I had surround sound turned on. When I realized that, I was just in love with how it made me feel. I was like, "Yeah, this is me. This is who I am." Cannabis is how the things in my life have evolved and how I've been able to achieve so many things.

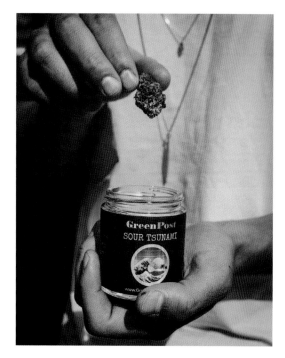

JW: Have you gone back to taking photos for yourself? Have you found the joy in it again?

KV: Yeah, I still do photography, but I'm really selective in what I do for money. On a daily basis, I do take pictures just for myself even if I don't share them with anyone. I think it's a part of me that's never gonna go away. It is something that I still offer for our clients. I'm really grateful that I'm still able to do that, but I also enjoy the freedom of not having to do it.

JW: The burnout is real! If you spend all day everyday using your camera for other people; it's hard to want to take it out for yourself. It's great that you found a way to do it for yourself again.

KV: For sure. It took a lot of effort. Dissolving the photography partnership wasn't easy. Leaving relationships that aren't benefiting you anymore is rough, but it needs to happen. I was on autopilot. So many of us are just walking around like we're asleep, but cannabis helped me stop, look up, be present, and ask myself, "Am I OK with everything in my life right now? Am I happy? Am I living the life I want?" I was pretty relentless at finding the clarity that I needed to level up. So I spent a year in seclusion, reading a lot, listening to audiobooks and podcasts, and just shutting myself in to find myself. Cannabis was with me through all of that.

JW: So for you, cannabis isn't just about feeling creative, it's helped you figure out who you are and what you want.

KV: Absolutely. And that's what led me to being in the industry. I realized that of all the people I knew, my friends, and my family, I was always the one who had an uncertain path because I was a freelancer. I was a self-employed entrepreneur. I tried doing different businesses, and even though I always succeeded, cannabis was a huge part of that success. But it was missing from the public eye. It was always a part of me, but it wasn't something I vocalized or something I advocated for.

In that disconnect, I realized I wasn't fully living my truth. I was in the cannabis closet. I felt like it had been really holding me back creatively and in business not being able to come out and say "Look, I smoke weed, but I'm still fucking badass." I decided to embrace it and be vocal about it and advocate for it. As soon as I decided that, that was when I landed my first client in the industry, photographing dispensaries and cultivation centers. Right away, I was like, "Yes, exactly. This is what I want to be doing. I wanna be surrounded by this all the time."

JW: Is smoking something you do specifically to get in the creative headspace, or do you just tend to smoke periodically, and creativity is a byproduct of that?

KV: Earlier in my life, I would say, probably the latter. I liked to smoke all day. Wake and bake and all that. Nowadays, I listen more to what my body and mind want and need. It's different every day. In his book, *The Cannabis Manifesto*, Steve DeAngelo emphasizes choosing cannabis for wellness and not for intoxication, so that's a principle I've put in place in my life. I try to approach it in that way. How can this enhance me as a person for what I need to achieve right now?

JW: Do you have particular creative rituals in your work?

KV: If I'm trying to create a logo or something like that for example, I do a brain dump on a piece of paper. Just literally just throw out whatever comes into my head, whatever image, whatever drawing, or whatever the pen or pencil wants me to do. I just spend 10 or 15 minutes doing that, dumping everything out, and then I can intentionally get to a space where I've cleared my head and I can focus on the best way forward.

In photography, it's similar because with film you can't be trigger happy. You have to have that decisive moment and decide when you're gonna take that shot. You compose it in your

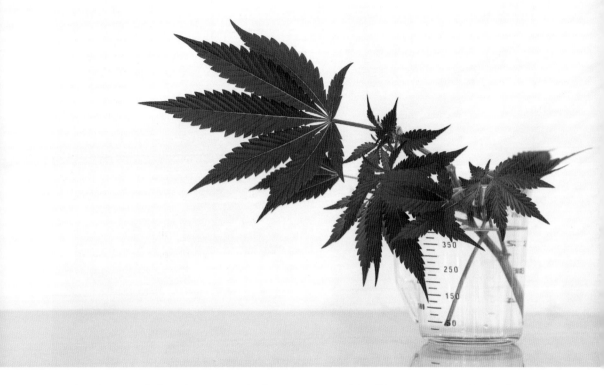

mind and get ready for it 'cause you don't want to waste film. Film is expensive. So I still approach it in that way. I take my time in composing the photo so that it's just one click and I got what I needed.

JW: Are there certain strains you prefer?

KV: If I can get my hands on it, White Widow is the ultimate strain for me. It's an indica-dominant strain, but I think because of the terpenes, it has uplifting creative effects, so I love it. I feel like I get a lot of stuff done when I'm on White Widow. Strawberry Cough is another one that's just so tasty. As far as concentrates, Super Lemon Haze. Oh my God; it smells so good. You want to drink it or eat it. I wanna put it on as perfume.

JW: Do you prefer smoking?

KV: I do like the ritual of smoking flower. I dabbled in dabbing, and I still do it sometimes, but with dabbing I have to plan stuff out. I can't do much for the rest of the day. I usually roll my own joints. I got really good at it when I went to Amsterdam in 2010. I was forced to learn because if you didn't want to get a pre-roll mixed with tobacco, you had to roll your own.

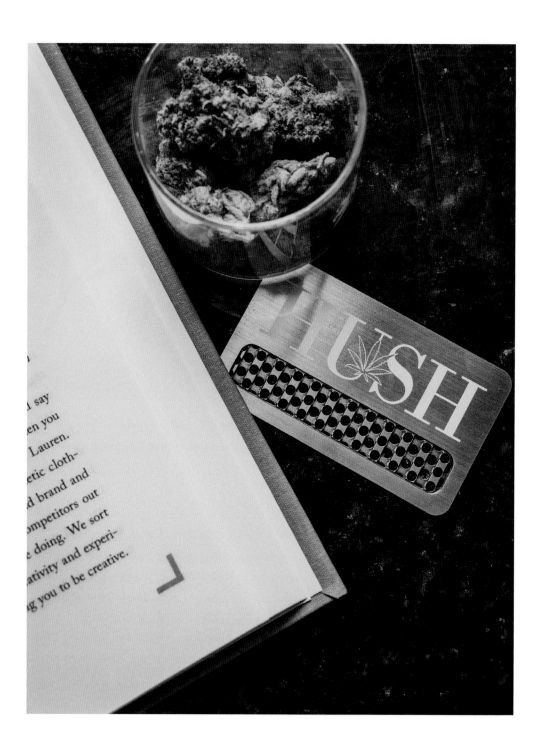

CANNABIS FOR CREATIVES

JW: Do you ever take edibles?

KV: I do! But I have a super low tolerance for edibles, and I've learned that the hard way. Savory edibles, I'm usually OK with, but with gummies or anything else that has sugar, my body metabolizes it really quickly. I get really high on a small, small dosage. Now, I've learned I need to microdose when it comes to edibles, so just like two and a half or five milligrams at a time.

JW: I'm the same way. The package will say a dose is something like 10 milligrams, and I'll bite a third of it off and just wait, because otherwise…I mean, I've been smoking since I was a teenager, so I know what I'm doing, but I can still have these unexpected edible experiences where I'm like, "Am I on mushrooms right now?"

KV: Exactly! It definitely hits those different receptors and gives you more of that psychedelic kind of high. I think I was high for three days one time, from just overconsuming. Some people can eat a 100-milligram bar of chocolate and be fine. Even more than that. For me, just like a milligram or two, and I'm good.

JW: Dialing out the work you do in the cannabis industry, how has the changing attitude and legal status of cannabis affected your creative relationship with it?

KV: I feel more confident in openly supporting something that's legalized, even in my personal life and sharing more about cannabis with my parents. Educating them and getting them to use CBD has been really impactful because if it wasn't legal, they would never be open to it. The illegality was their whole perception. They knew I smoked pot. I got caught so many times as a kid, but to them it was just like, "It's illegal, and that's all that matters." So now that the whole perception has shifted, it's been positive for me personally.

JW: It does seem like the world is lining up for you as far as the things you care about and the talents you can bring to the table in your company. It seems like you're living your best life.

KV: I'm not quite there yet, but I'm on my way. It took a long time to get to this place and a lot of relearning and reprogramming myself. That's gonna be a lifetime journey, but I'm glad to be where I am and that I found it. I appreciate that cannabis was a huge, huge part of it. Just like certain songs remind you of breakups or sad days or happy days. I have the same experience with cannabis. It's been a really good companion and support system for me to have that security of, "You know what? Everything's gonna be fine. No matter how it turns out."

JW: If you couldn't imbibe cannabis at all, would that throw a wrench in your creative process?

KV: I don't think so, because I remember having those really creative moments without using cannabis. I think being on it enhances what's already there. I don't think it makes you better or worse; it just enhances you. It brings you to a different space where you see things differently. It also helps you see when you're wrong or when something is a bad idea; it helps with that clarity and truth.

JW: Can you describe what it feels like when you smoke and have that creative enhancement?

KV: When I'm high? I don't know if I've ever described it!

JW: It's hard to put into words, right?

KV: It is! OK…I think once it hits, and it depends whether that's an edible 45 minutes later or just a few minutes after you smoke a joint, but when it hits, like Bob Marley said: you feel no pain. Whatever you were stressed about, whatever thoughts were consuming you, things that you were worried about, things that were making you anxious…it goes away. You get a different perspective about what you really should be focusing on, which is the present moment. When I'm high, that's what it triggers in my brain. They call it high because, to me, you are on this higher level, a higher dimension, a higher perspective, where you're able to see what really matters, and it's pretty simple. We tend to complicate things when our thoughts are consuming us, but once you're high, you're just more aware and more in touch with the things around you. You notice and appreciate things that you wouldn't normally pay attention to.

JW: It sounds like a superpower when you describe it that way. Elevated living.

KV: I know! I had a successful photography business, and 99% of that time I was high. You can't tell me that cannabis consumers can't be successful entrepreneurs. People are finally coming into the open about it, so it's easier to find people who are more aligned with you. I was able to build a completely new network of friends and a new support system of people who are also into cannabis. They're working towards the same thing that we're working towards, so it's been really great. It makes me really happy.

CHAPTER 6

EXPLORING YOUR OWN CREATIVITY WITH CANNABIS

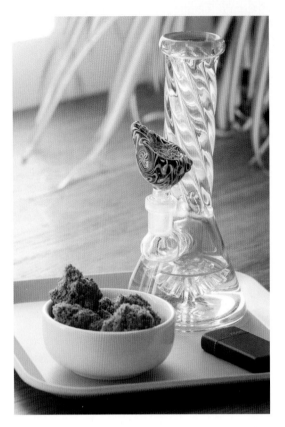

You might have already suspected just how individual the creative experience tends to be. As we've seen in the preceding interviews, no two artists are alike. The type of work artists create, the environments they require, the places they search for inspiration, and the methods they use to stay engaged and motivated: these variables are what makes them unique, giving their work impact and resonance. But the creative experience is fluid. Just as methods and values vary from artist to artist, techniques and processes adapt and change within an artist's lifetime. Things that once worked before may not work again.

In cultivating our own creative environments, both physical and mental, we've all experienced the frustration of a fickle muse. When she doesn't show up, we may push ourselves harder, or we may shut down. The path through requires work. After learning about such a beautifully varied collection of creators, you may feel inspired to explore some of the techniques that work for them. You may want to head over to the dispensary and start experimenting. Before you do, it will help to reflect on your own creative experiences thus far.

In his book *The Mirror Thief*, Martin Seay presented a statement that really resonated with me and my desire to study and understand creativity. He wrote, "The explorer who reaches a summit and curses to find another's ice-axe already there is no explorer at all, but only a conqueror and a thug. Every worthwhile initiative is a collaboration, a conspiracy, a series of coded messages passed across the years from hand to anonymous hand."

We don't develop our sense of creativity in a vacuum. There are always influences, be they social, chemical, or inspirational. We grow from the insights of others as we explore and reach new summits in our art. So, I invite you to join the conversation. Discover your own insights that will someday help you play a part in someone else's creative investigations.

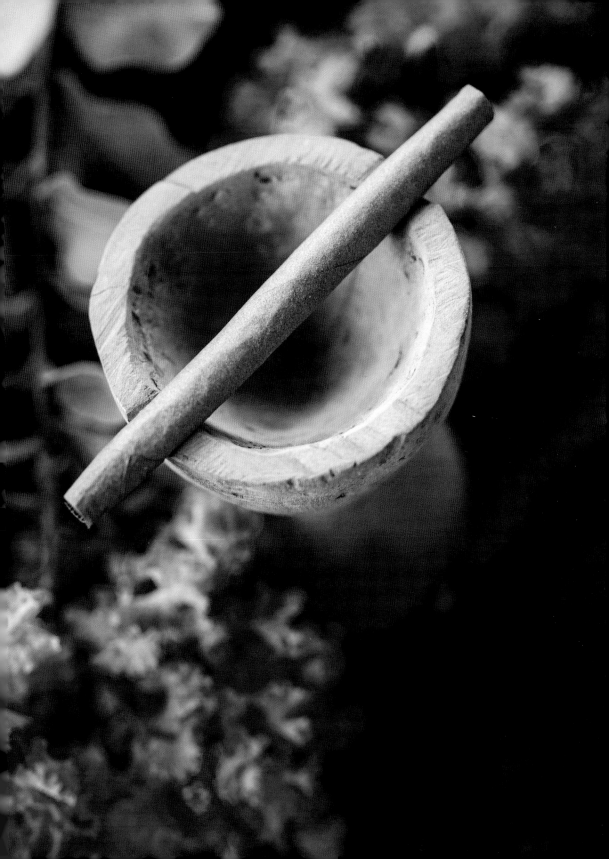

To get the most out of the following section, I recommend starting a "Cannabis and Creativity" journal (or just a "Creativity" journal, if you're not quite ready to experiment with pot). Personal reflections about our experiences can help guide us toward more actionable paths of creation. You are the next case study adding to this research. So, consider grabbing a notebook or starting a file on your computer to track your experiences, stoned or sober, creative or creatively frustrated, and everything in between.

Find Your Own Creative Goldilocks Zone

Finding the creative Goldilocks Zone is a vital piece of the puzzle. You may have already developed a system that seems to work for you. You may have put a great deal of thought into it, or you might approach it casually from a "what feels right, right now" perspective.

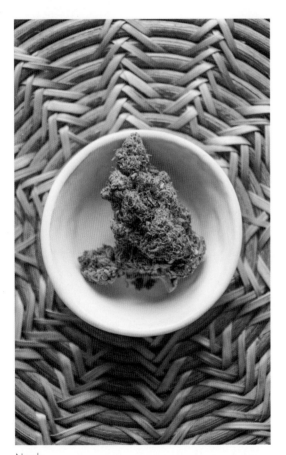

Nerds

Regardless of how we've gotten there, we've all had a creative epiphany at some point in our lives. Think back to a time when you had a total "Aha!" moment. Maybe you came up with the perfect phrase for a poem or a song. Maybe you felt that undeniable impulse to physically create a painting or a recipe. Maybe you looked at the vista before you and just knew how to frame it into a photograph.

What did that look like for you? In each interview, I asked artists to tell me about their artistic journeys. Think back to your journey. Consider your earliest creative moments in childhood or the standout experiences in your life that helped you find a love for the act of creating. What were those experiences? What story would you tell me in an interview about your life as a creative and how you got to where you are today? How would you describe your current creative process? What creative rituals do you employ?

As you explore your history as a creative person, look for clues in your past processes that help you better understand your ideal creative Goldilocks Zone. Do you create better when you're alone? Was your best creation related to the expansive imagination and lack of boundaries found in childhood? Do you feel more inspired by new places or familiar haunts? Is there a time of day that seems to call your creative energy forward? Are you inspired by bustling cities, or landscapes in the wilderness?

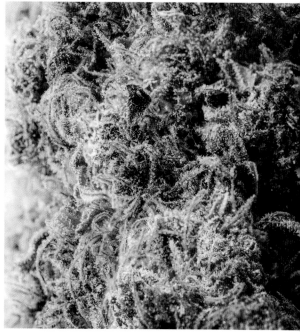

Nerds

We've heard from artists who need music, who prefer to be energized by exercise, and some who need to work within a relaxed, meditative state. What has your creative Goldilocks Zone looked like in the past? How can you recapture those energies or grow from those prior experiences to help call your creativity forward in the future?

Write it all down. Every insight is a step toward more productive creativity.

Explore Your Past Cannabis Experiences

I'm fairly certain that you, the readers of this book, will cover the full spectrum of cannabis use, from those who've never tried it, to those who enjoy cannabis on an all-day everyday basis. Maybe it was more of a social thing in your youth but now, with all of the changing legislation, you're curious about exploring pot again. Maybe psychoactive elements like THC are outside of your comfort zone, and you're more interested in trying CBD.

No matter your history of cannabis use, you don't have to justify your comfort level or preferences to anyone. If you're not interested in THC or even CBD, you'll get no peer

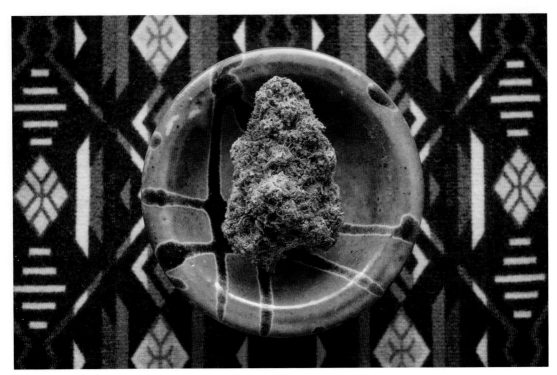

Snowcap

pressure from me. But if you have enjoyed pot in the past, or possibly tried it and not found it enjoyable, let's dig a little deeper into your experiences.

When did cannabis come into your life? How did you first experience it? Were you one of the many members of the population who didn't really get high the first time around? Did you completely overdo it and fall asleep or get paranoid or eat a whole pizza in one sitting?

Explore your memories of cannabis in various eras of your life. If you used to take more pleasure in it than you do now, try to figure out what's changed. Is it about your environment or how you imbibe? Is it a question of doing it alone versus with friends or at a party? Have you found more comfort and less paranoia in legalized areas? Does legality matter to you? Do you judge yourself for when, how, or why you choose to get high?

I'm not a psychologist, nor do I play one on TV, but I am a hyper-introspective person. High or clear minded, I'm always searching for the reasoning behind my emotions, behavior, successes, and failures. If your mind works this way, too, asking yourself these questions will feel fairly normal. If you're a stranger to self-analysis, these pursuits may take a bit more work. It's worth it. One common thread among all of the interviews you read in this book is that each of these artists and cannabis enthusiasts have personally explored their experiences in depth to better understand what effects cannabis has on their lives. These artists can refer to the cannabis high in terminology that best suits their experience because they've spent plenty of time thinking about it. Whether you call it a head change, a slight hum, a spirit flight, letting out the balloons, adding contrast, or something else, ask yourself:

- Do you believe cannabis makes you more creative?
- When or how did you discover that cannabis could affect your creative process?
- Do you imbibe when you tend to create or is it an occasional byproduct?
- Why do you think cannabis makes you more creative? Or, why don't you?
- What does the cannabis-inspired creative energy feel like?

By answering these questions, you can start to draw out the similarities in your experiences, determine what beneficial results cannabis can have on your creative workflow, and hopefully harness some of these concepts to work toward more productive and sustainable cannabis-fueled creative experiences in the future.

Track Your Cannabis Experiences

Having performed some reflective work on your past and present as a creative and/or cannabis enthusiast, your future experimentation with strains, methods of getting high, dosage, and terpene profiles will benefit from some organizational tracking. Because we're still at least a few years away from actionable research in the genetics of cannabis and its related neurological effects on us, we're all still in the same trial-and-error experimentation boat. Just like wine enthusiasts keep tasting notes about different vintages and expressions, cannabis lovers can keep our

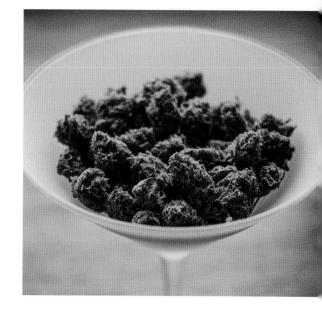

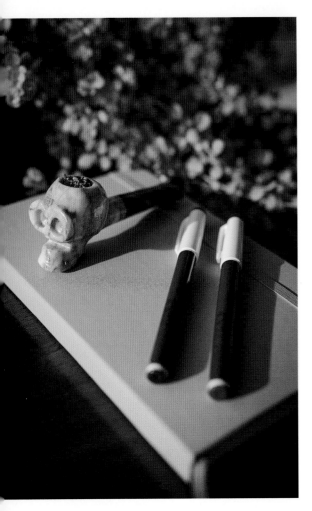

own records of what we experience. So, as you work your way through what the dispensary offers, consider keeping track of what you try and the experiences it inspires.

One quick disclaimer to note: cannabis is still federally illegal in the United States and many other countries around the world. The chances of the FBI or DEA knocking on your door and seizing your "Cannabis and Creativity" notebook to use against you are probably slim, but you might secretly be a modern-day Pablo Escobar or something, and I have no way of knowing. In any case, it's generally a good idea to be as discreet as possible about what the Feds still consider use of an illegal drug. Maybe don't leave your cannabis notes on your work computer. If you aren't buying your pot in a legal dispensary, err on the side of not incriminating other people or yourself. I'm also not advising you to enjoy cannabis illegally. I hate that I have to say that, but here we are. Write a letter to your senator or the president. Donate money to advocacy groups. Vote. Someday, we'll get to release a new edition of this book that will say on the very first page: "Hey, pot is legal in the US now! Good for us. We deserve it, so smoke it if you've got it." That day is not today.

That said, here's one helpful way to organize your notes. Include as much or as little of it as you feel comfortable.

Cannabis and Tasting Experience Notes

Strain: Include information about the name of the strain and the parent strains when possible. This will make it easier to find similar strains that you might also like. *(Example: Blue Dream. Parents: Blueberry and Haze)*

Dispensary: We know that one dispensary's version of a strain may vary genetically from another, so it helps to record the specific dispensary. *(Example: Silver Stem)*

Category: Is it listed as indica, sativa, or hybrid? While we know that these terms don't necessarily indicate what sort of experience you'll have, they are helpful to track. You'll start to see if you gravitate toward one category or another. *(Example: sativa-dominant hybrid)*

Scent and flavor: You can include terpenes listed on the packaging, but your experience is the focus here, so what flavors and scents do you notice? Do you like the smell and flavor? Are they subtle or strong? Is it citrusy, earthy, or something else? *(Example: fruity, earthy, and floral)*

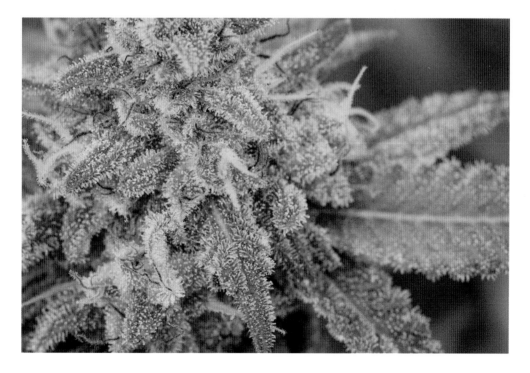

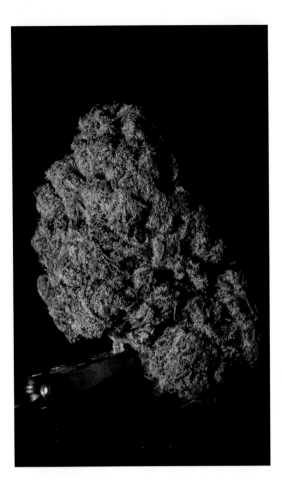

Physical appearance: Is it a compact bud? A wispy one? Lots of seeds or very clean? Red hairs? Trichomes? Is it green? Purple? Yellow? *(Example: green and purple, compact, dense bud with plenty of red hairs)*

Method of imbibing: Did you smoke it in a pipe or bong? Roll it in a joint or blunt? Eat it in a gummy or vape it? We know that how we get high has a lot to do with the effects, so track the differences if you smoke it one day and vape it the next. *(Example: pre-roll cone)*

Dosage: Does the packaging list THC or CBD percentage? Track any active cannabinoids listed. If it's an edible, how much did you ingest over what period of time, and how long did it take to hit? If it's flower, how much did you smoke? *(Example: 18% THC, 1 gram smoked in a single session)*

Effects: Body high, head high, or both? Sleepy or euphoric? Did you laugh a lot or get serious and introspective? Did you move through multiple effects over the course of your high? What were they? *(Example: relaxed body high combined with heightened attention and creative energy)*

Notes: This is where you get as specific as you want. Reflect on what you feel. Do you like it? Do you feel more creative? Do you want to fall asleep or go on a neighborhood walkabout or eat everything in your fridge? Are you paranoid, excited, calm, or reflective? Did you paint for six hours or write for two? You can also take your notes beyond the strain and high and just reflect on your current creative life, your hopes, dreams, feelings, etc. If you were already having a stressed-out day, and pot calmed you down, note it. If you got more stressed or anxious, note that too.

CANNABIS FOR CREATIVES

CONTINUING THE CYCLE OF CREATIVITY

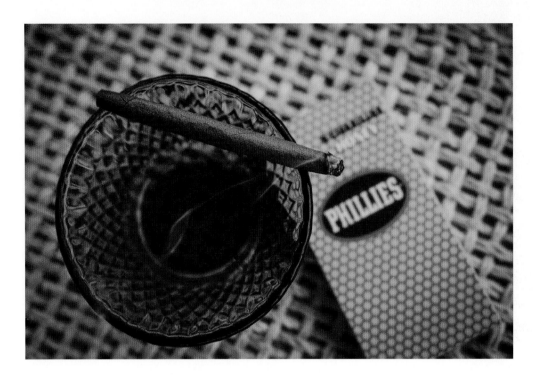

Well, we've been on quite the journey. We've learned about the ways that humans have been utilizing cannabis for thousands of years to advance religion, medicine, commerce, industry, and more. We've explored the complicated relationship between legality and cultural use and addressed some of the very real, very unfortunate discriminatory practices that laid the foundation for cannabis's illegality in the United States. We've talked about the plant itself, how it's grown, how it's bred, and how it's been shaped by human intervention. We've discussed all of the complications surrounding studying creativity itself, let alone cannabis-fueled creativity. We've ventured into the neuroscience of cannabis and how and why it affects us. We've met a wonderful collection of artists and heard all about their creative journeys and experiences with cannabis. Finally, we've taken all of that information and started thinking about how we can enhance and sustain our own creative pursuits and inspiration.

Even though we've done all that, we've only begun the conversation. Cannabis and creativity are both topics that you could explore for a lifetime and still find amazing new things to learn. Through the passage of time, as cultural and legal regulations and misconceptions continue to relax and abate, I'm certain that more and more big-C Creatives and little-c creatives alike will come out of the cannabis closet and share their stories, insights, and what

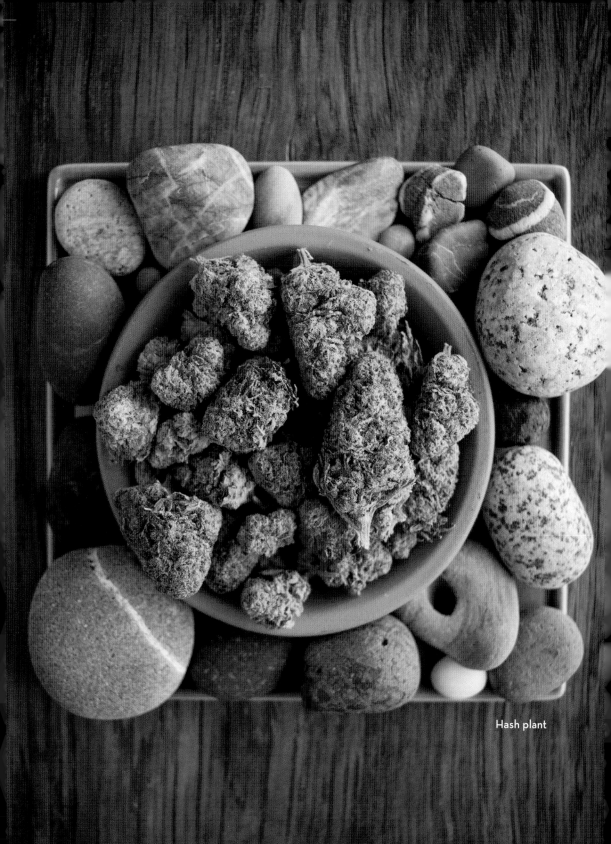

Hash plant

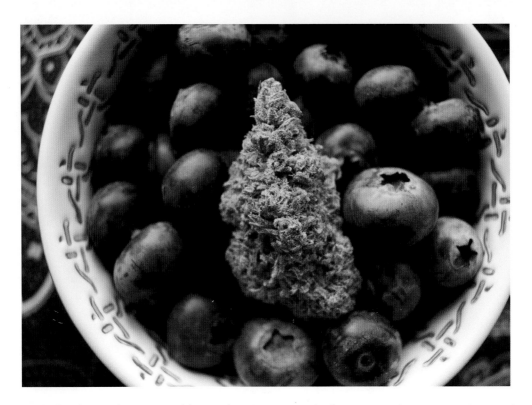

works for them. I, for one, would never have put so much of my personal experience into these pages even five years ago. Imagine what it will be like five years from now.

Cannabis's legitimacy as a medicinal and creative tool can only continue to grow. I can't wait to see what else we will learn about this magic plant in the not too distant future. Whether you're an enthusiast, canna-curious, or just looking for a new way of thinking about creativity, thank you for joining me on this exploration with an open mind. As a novelist, journalist, and someone who was preoccupied with understanding and exploring creativity, Arthur Koestler expressed, "Creativity is a type of learning process where the teacher and pupil are located in the same individual."

In writing this book, I've been the teacher, the pupil, and at times, the guidance counselor. Now it's your turn to teach, learn, and explore. So, in the words of Cypress Hill, "Roll it up, light it up, smoke it up, inhale, exhale."

GLOSSARY

Blunt: A cigar or cigarillo that has been emptied of tobacco and filled with cannabis.

Bong: A variety of cannabis pipe that filters the smoke through water for a smoother hit. Bongs can be made of glass, plastic, wood, ceramic, or a variety of other materials.

Bowl: A commonly used name for a cannabis pipe.

Cannabinoids: Chemical compounds found in cannabis. They can be psychoactive or non-psychoactive.

Dab Rig: A smoking setup similar to a bong used to smoke oil, rosin, shatter, wax, or other varieties of cannabis concentrates. The act of using a dab rig is called "dabbing."

Ditch-weed: Wild growing or feral cannabis often found in former hemp producing areas. Colloquially, ditch-weed describes cannabis of poor quality or containing very little THC.

Dooby: Another name for a *joint*.

Edible: A candy, baked good, savory treat, beverage, or other ingestible item that has been infused with cannabinoids.

Endocannabinoid System: The body's complex natural system for nerve signaling to maintain vital elements of bodily functioning.

Hashish: A resinous extract of the cannabis plant featuring concentrated cannabinoids and terpenes. Also called hash.

Hemp: A non-psychoactive member of the cannabis family.

Hookah: A water pipe with one or more flexible tube mouthpieces used for smoking cannabis and/or tobacco.

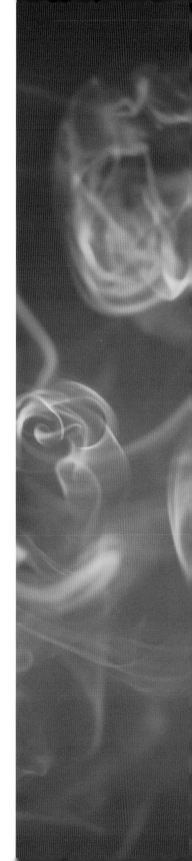

Hotboxing: The act of filling an enclosed space like a closet or bathroom with large quantities of cannabis smoke.

Joint: A paper cigarette containing cannabis.

Kief: A fine dust composed of loose cannabis trichomes.

Landrace Strain: A strain of cannabis that has proliferated in relative isolation without crossbreeding, allowing it to remain pure. These are some of the earliest documented strains of cannabis.

Microdosing: The act of taking very small amounts of cannabis or other substances for a diluted effect.

Moonrocks: Cannabis flower dipped in hash oil and rolled in cannabis kief.

Psychotropic: A chemical substance that can alter mood, behavior, perception, or cognition.

Spliff: A joint filled with a mixture of cannabis and tobacco.

Sploof: A paper towel tube filled with dryer sheets used to mask the smell of exhaled cannabis smoke.

Steamroller: A large cannabis pipe consisting of a hollow tube and a bowl at one end used for taking very large hits.

THC: Tetrahydrocannabinol, the primary psychoactive cannabinoid in cannabis.

Trichomes: Tiny mushroom shaped appendages found on cannabis flowers that contain high concentrations of terpenes and cannabinoids.

Vaporizer: A smoking device that heats cannabis flower, oil, or resin to a controlled temperature without combustion for a smoother smoke.

Volcano: A brand of vaporizer that involves filling a plastic bag with a quantity of vaporized cannabis.

Wax: A high potency cannabis concentrate that can be used in a dab rig or smoked on top of a bowl of ground cannabis flower.

TEXT REFERENCES AND IMAGE CITATIONS

All images in chapter 5 courtesy of the artists. Individual photo credits, where known, are provided below:

Page 103: Photo by Jeff Wilson Photography

Page 104: Photo by Nathan Edge

Pages 182–184: Photos by Alan Hess

Pages 204–210: Photos by Kay Villamin

Page 11: https://publicdomainreview.org/collection/miniatures-from-a-12th-century-medical-and-herbal-collection.

Page 14 (right image): Gottlieb, William P. Portrait of Billie Holiday and Mister, Downbeat, New York, N.Y., ca. Feb. 1947. Monographic. Photograph. https://www.loc.gov/item/gottlieb.04281/.

Page 14 (left image): Gottlieb, William P. Portrait of Louis Armstrong, Aquarium, New York, N.Y., ca. July 1946. Monographic. Photograph. https://www.loc.gov/item/gottlieb.00231/.

Page 15: Allan, Ted. MGM photo of Groucho Marx from *A Day at the Races*, April 1, 1937. Photograph. https://commons.wikimedia.org/wiki/File:Groucho_Marx_A_Day_at_the_Races.jpg.

Page 19: illustrations sourced from the University of Iowa Library's Digital Collection

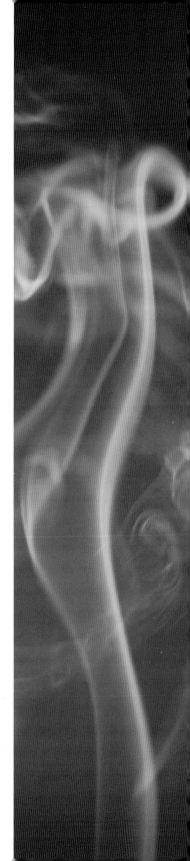

Bibliography

Advokat, Claire D., et al. *Julien's Primer of DRUG Action: A Comprehensive Guide to the Actions, Uses, and Side Effects of Psychoactive Drugs*. New York: Worth Publishers, 2019.

Bigthink. *The Neuroscience of Genius, Creativity, and Improvisation, with Heather Berlin*. YouTube, 4 Mar. 2015, www.youtube.com/watch?v=4anaU6rdU1Q.

Black, Bobby, et al. "'Easy Rider' Peter Fonda Returns to Pot in New Film." *Cannabis Now*, 7 Aug. 2018, cannabisnow.com/easy-rider-peter-fonda-returns-to-pot-in-new-film/.

Breathes, William. "Cannabis Time CAPSULE, 1948: Robert Mitchum's Marijuana Bust." *Westword*, 22 June 2021, www.westword.com/news/cannabis-time-capsule-1948-robert-mitchums-marijuana-bust-6052085.

Brenan, Megan. "Support for Legal Marijuana Inches up to New High of 68%." Gallup.com, Gallup, 23 Mar. 2021, news.gallup.com/poll/323582/support-legal-marijuana-inches-new-high.aspx.

Cantor, Hallie. "Groucho Marx Entertained the Troops with Weed Jokes in 1943." *Vulture*, 19 Dec. 2011, www.vulture.com/2011/12/groucho-marx-entertained-the-troops-with-weed-jokes-in-1943.html.

Chen, Angus. "Some of the Parts: Is Marijuana's 'Entourage EFFECT' Scientifically Valid?" *Scientific American*, 20 Apr. 2017, www.scientificamerican.com/article/some-of-the-parts-is-marijuana-rsquo-s-ldquo-entourage-effect-rdquo-scientifically-valid/.

Donahue, Michelle. "Earliest Evidence for Cannabis Smoking Discovered in Ancient Tombs." *Culture News*, National Geographic, 12 June 2019, www.nationalgeographic.com/culture/article/earliest-evidence-cannabis-marijuana-smoking-china-tombs#:~:text=The%20earliest%20direct%20evidence%20for,in%20the%20journal%20Science%20Advances.

Dumas, Alexandre, 1802-1870. *The Count of Monte Cristo*. New York: Penguin Books, 2001.

Earleywine, Mitchell. *Understanding Marijuana: A New Look at the Scientific Evidence*. Oxford: Oxford University Press, 2002.

The Equity Organization. "Our Vision." The Equity Organization, equityorganization.org/war-on-drugs.

Freeman, Tom P., et al. "Cannabis Dampens the Effects of Music in Brain Regions Sensitive to Reward and Emotion." *International Journal of Neuropsychopharmacology*, vol. 21, issue 1 (2018): 21-32. doi:10.1093/ijnp/pyx082.

Ginsberg, Allen. "The Great Marijuana Hoax." *The Atlantic Monthly*, Nov. 1966, pp. 104–114.

Hand, Andrew, Alexa Blake, Paul Kerrigan, Phineas Samuel, and Jeremy Friedberg. "History of medical cannabis." Cannabis: Medical Aspects, no. 9 (2016): 387–394.

HERODOTUS. *The Histories*. Edited by Paul Cartledge. Translated by Tom Holland, Penguin Classics, 2014.

Kaufman, Scott Barry. "The Neuroscience of Creativity: A Q&A with Anna Abraham." *Scientific American Blog Network*, Scientific American, 4 Jan. 2019, blogs.scientificamerican.com/beautiful-minds/the-neuroscience-of-creativity-a-q-a-with-anna-abraham/.

King, Stephen. *Everything's Eventual: 14 Dark Tales*. New York: Scribner, 2018.

Kleon, Austin. *Keep Going: 10 Ways to Stay Creative in Good Times and Bad*. New York: Workman Publishing, 2019.

Koontz, Alison, and Marianne Bronner. "The Circuitry of Creativity: How Our Brains Innovate Thinking." *Caltech Letters*, 12 Mar. 2019, caltechletters.org/science/what-is-creativity.

Kossen, Jeremy. "How Does Cannabis Consumption Affect the Brain?" *Leafly*, 28 July 2020, www.leafly.com/news/health/how-marijuana-affects-the-brain.

Kowal, Mikael A., et al. "Cannabis and creativity: highly potent cannabis impairs divergent thinking in regular cannabis users." *Psychopharmacology* vol. 232,6 (2015): 1123-34. doi:10.1007/s00213-014-3749-1.

LaFrance, Emily M. and Carrie Cuttler. "Inspired by Mary Jane? Mechanisms underlying enhanced creativity in cannabis users." *Consciousness and Cognition* vol. 56 (2017): 68-76. doi:10.1016/j.concog.2017.10.009.

Laursen, L. Botany: The cultivation of weed. *Nature* 525, S4–S5 (2015). https://doi.org/10.1038/525S4a.

Lee, Martin A. Smoke Signals: A Social History of Marijuana—Medical, Recreational and Scientific. New York: Scribner, 2013.

Lockie, Alex. "Top Nixon Adviser Reveals the Racist Reason He Started the 'War on Drugs' Decades Ago." *Business Insider*, 31 July 2019, www.businessinsider.com/ nixon-adviser-ehrlichman-anti-left-anti-black-war-on-drugs-2019-7.

McKenna, Terence. *Food of the Gods the Search for the Original Tree of Knowledge*. London: Ebury Publishing, 2010.

Piomelli, D., and Ethan B. Russo. (2016) The Cannabis sativa versus Cannabis indica debate: an interview with Ethan Russo, MD, Cannabis and Cannabinoid Research 1:1, 44–46, DOI: 10.1089/can.2015.29003.ebr.

Russo, Ethan B. "Taming THC: potential cannabis synergy and phytocannabinoid-terpenoid entourage effects." *British Journal of Pharmacology* vol. 163,7 (2011): 1344-64. doi:10.1111/j.1476-5381.2011.01238.x.

Russo, Ethan B. "The Case for the Entourage Effect and Conventional Breeding of Clinical Cannabis: No 'Strain,' No Gain." *Frontiers in Plant Science* vol. 9 1969. 9 Jan. 2019, doi:10.3389/fpls.2018.01969.

Sawler, Jason et al. "The Genetic Structure of Marijuana and Hemp." *PloS one* vol. 10,8 e0133292. 26 Aug. 2015, doi:10.1371/journal.pone.0133292.

Schafer, Gráinne, et al. "Investigating the interaction between schizotypy, divergent thinking and cannabis use." *Consciousness and Cognition* 21.1 (2012): 292-298.

Seay, Martin. *The Mirror Thief: A Novel*. New York: Melville House, 2017.

Vergara, Daniela, et al. "Genomic Evidence That Governmentally Produced Cannabis Sativa Poorly Represents Genetic Variation Available in State Markets." *BioRxiv*, Cold Spring Harbor Laboratory, 1 Jan. 2021, www.biorxiv.org/content/10.1101/2021.02.13.431041v1.

Weil, Andrew. *The Natural Mind*. New York: Penguin, 1975.

Weiner, Eric. *The Geography of Genius: A Search for the World's Most Creative Places from Ancient Athens to Silicon Valley*. New York: Simon and Schuster, 2016.

Zinberg, Norman E. *Drug, Set, and Setting: The Basis for Controlled Intoxicant Use*. New Haven: Yale University Press, 1984. Print.

ACKNOWLEDGMENTS

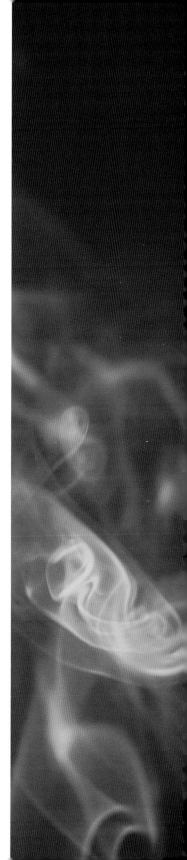

Bringing this book into being involved many intelligent, creative, talented, and giving people and I so appreciate their generous help and support!

I relied heavily on the assistance of a few fabulous experts. Dr. Jeremy Teissere provided an energetic crash course on neuroscience and cannabis, and recommended many of my most useful published sources. Dr. Josh Kaplan was an invaluable resource for getting up to date with contemporary research in neuroscience. He also graciously reviewed the neuroscience sections of the book. He was an enormous help and I'm very appreciative of his expertise and his willingness to advise me as a total random who emailed him out of the blue! Thanks to Ellen Herschel who is studying neuroscience and creativity as a graduate student at the University of Southern California, and who answered so many of my questions and made great source recommendations for the study of creativity. Ezra Huscher provided enormous insight into the botany and genomics of cannabis, through a lengthy video chat and numerous follow-up emails, and I can't thank him enough!

Thanks to the friends and colleagues who shared my interview requests far and wide and made introductions to interview subjects. Among them are Jay Dusard, Anna Young, Alan Hess (who also allowed the use of his images), Sara Clausnitzer, Stephen Wooten, and Mary Pat Bergmann. You folks made this book richer through your connections and I so appreciate you! Maria Ivey and Ellie Newman who made the interview with Ray Benson possible, thank you so much for your help!

Thanks to the Rocky Nook team: Scott Cowlin for taking the plunge on a book that was probably just a bit outside RN's comfort zone, Ted Waitt for being such an encouraging and helpful resource through all portions of book development, Jocelyn Howell for being a fabulous editor and a stellar human being (I'm always happy to see your name in my inbox), Mercedes Murray for coaxing me to pitch the book and offering suggestions for finding interview subjects, and all of the other fabulous RN folks who work tirelessly to bring fantastic books into the world.

Paul Good, thank you for chasing down models to get signed releases! Nelson Ruger, my dear friend, thank you for creating an enchanting cover design. Working with you creatively is one of my favorite things on this planet! Thanks to Jake Flaherty for the fabulous interior design. It's such a beautiful book. My enormous gratitude to John McAmis who took my somewhat vague requests for illustrations and ran with them as only he could.

I want to thank the wonderful collection of artists who trusted me to tell their stories. I am inspired by your passion for your work and your willingness to tell the world about cannabis's value in your lives. Juerg Federer, Kenton Williams, Anna Pollock, TJ Kennedy, Trisha Smith, Sanjay Patel, Nikki Barber, Dariusz Malysa, Daniela Valdez, Kael Mendoza, Christopher O'Riley, Gary Wingfield Jr., Bruno Wu, Cara Dilluvio, Barrett Guzaldo, Richard Magarin, Mark Karan, Kay Villamin, Colton Clifford, Michael Marras, Garrett Shore, Amanda Hosking, Carlos Mandelaveitia, Mark McDowell, Nelson Ruger, and Ray Benson, thank you for your time, for your insights, and for sharing your work with me! To the artists who preferred anonymity, I so appreciate your willingness to share your experiences and the trust you placed in me to keep your confidence.

Thanks to my personal cheering section, a wonderful cohort of supportive friends and family: Brandan, Emily, Rachel, Adam, Matt, Abby, my in-laws Mike and Sharon Wright, and my brother Joshua Boydstun who fields non-stop and potentially mind-numbing grammar and punctuation questions. To my parents Robert and Suzanne Boydstun, who are not cannabis people but have always supported and respected cannabis's place in my life, thank you for everything you do and have done to help me develop into an inquisitive, adventurous, and creative human being.

Finally, the greatest thanks belong to my husband and best friend, Cassius Wright, to whom this book is dedicated. I am the luckiest person in the world to have a partner in life who believes I'm capable of basically anything, encourages me to take on enormous challenges, and happily keeps me supplied with meals, snacks, fresh smoothies, and freshly packed bongs during long writing binges. This book, like most everything in my life, was possible because of your loving support.

INDEX

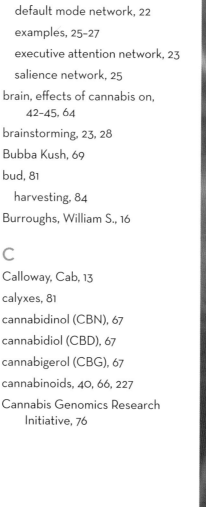

1960s, 16–18
1970s, 16–18
1980s, 18
2-AG, 41

A
acknowledgments, 233–234
activist, 149–151
actors, cannabis and, 15
Alternate Uses Task (AUT), 28
Anandamide, 41
anatomy, cannabis, 78
Anslinger, Harry J., 14
anti-inflammatory, 69
anxiety, cannabis and, 45, 67, 68
Armstrong, Louis, 13
aroma, cannabis, 68
art director, 117–123
artistic applications, history of, 11–20
autoflowering, 82

B
Barber, Nikki, 56, 157–163
Basie, William James "Count," 13
Beatles, the, 19
Benson, Ray, 100–106
Berry White, 68
biases, 37

Biggie Smalls, 18
blood pressure, 67
Blue Dream, 69
blunt, 227
bong, 227
bowl, 227
bracts, 81
brain networks, 22–26
    default mode network, 22
    examples, 25–27
    executive attention network, 23
    salience network, 25
brain, effects of cannabis on, 42–45, 64
brainstorming, 23, 28
Bubba Kush, 69
bud, 81
    harvesting, 84
Burroughs, William S., 16

C
Calloway, Cab, 13
calyxes, 81
cannabidinol (CBN), 67
cannabidiol (CBD), 67
cannabigerol (CBG), 67
cannabinoids, 40, 66, 227
Cannabis Genomics Research Initiative, 76

cannabis plant, 66–92
  anatomy, 78
  cannabinoids, 40, 66–67, 227
  clones, 85
  genome, 76–78
  growing, 74, 78–87
  harvesting, 84
  indica, 73
  landrace strains, 75
  names, 71–75
  sativa, 73
  trains, 68–75
  terpenes, 68–69
Cannatonic, 69
Carlin, George, 19
caryophyllene, 69
Cassady, Neal, 16
CB1/CB2 receptors, 41
Chappelle, Dave, 19
Cheech & Chong, 18
chefs, 95–99, 175–179
Chem Dog, 69
China, cannabis and, 10
Clifford, Colton, 186–190
Clift, Montgomery, 15
Clinton, George, 18
clones, growing from, 85
Club des Hashischins, 12
cola, 81
composer, 124–128
convergent thinking, 29–30
Cotton Candy Kush, 69
cotyledon, 80

counterculture movements, 16–18
creativity, 2–3
  brain networks and, 22–26
  cannabis and, 4–8, 33–38
  convergent thinking, 29–30
  divergent thinking, 28
  measuring after cannabis use, 30–32
  measuring, 28–32
  qualitative research, 33–38
  study of, 22–38
  testing, 28–30
Curtis, Tony, 15
Cypress Hill, 18

D

dab rig, 227
Dalí, Salvador, 19
de Balzac, Honoré, 12
de Nerval, Gérard, 12
Dean, James, 15
default mode network, 22
Delacroix, Eugène, 12
delta-8 THC, 66
delta-9 THC, 66
designers, 142–148
Dilluvio, Cara, 48, 52
ditch-weed, 227
divergent thinking, 28–29
Do-Si-Dos, 68
dooby, 227
Dope Chief, 164–168
dosage, 49–54
Dr. Dre, 18

drag, 186–190

Dumas, Alexandre, 12

Dylan, Bob, 19

E

Earleywine, Mitch, 34, 59

early use, 10

Easy Rider, 16

edibles, 88, 227

Ehrlichman, John, 18

Ellington, Duke, 13

endocannabinoid receptors, 41

endocannabinoid system, 40, 43, 227

endocannabinoids, 41

Entourage Effect, 70

epilepsy, treatment of, 67

excitatory neurons, 44

executive attention network, 23

exploration, personal, 214–222

F

fan leaves, 80

Federal Bureau of Narcotics, 14

federal prohibition of cannabis, 15, 220

Federer, Juerg "Fed," 62, 92, 95–99

Flaubert, Gustave, 12

flavor, cannabis, 68

flower, 81

flowering stage, 82

focus, 24

Fonda, Peter, 16

G

Gautier, Pierre Jules Theophile, 12

genome, cannabis, 76–78

Ginsberg, Allen, 16

Girl Scout Cookies, 69

glaucoma, treatment of, 67

glossary, 227–228

Goldilocks Zone, 49–54, 216–217

Grape Ape, 69

growing cannabis, 74, 78–87

   advanced, 85

   clones, 85

   indoor vs outdoor, 84

   stages, 82–83

Guzaldo, Barrett, 169–174

H

harvesting buds, 84

hash, 12, 227

Hashish Club, 12

Hemingway, Ernest, 19

hemp, 71, 227

Hendrix, Jimi, 19

high, controlling, 49

hip-hop, 18

history of cannabis use, 10–20

Holiday, Billie, 13

Hollywood, cannabis and, 15

hookah, 227

Hopper, Dennis, 16

Hosking, Amanda, 47, 63

hotboxing, 228

Hugo, Victor, 12

humidity, 84

humulene, 69

Hunter, Nathaniel C., 90, 149–151

Huscher, Ezra, 76

Hush Chicago, 203

I

imagination, 22

imbibing, different methods of, 87

indica, 73

inhibitory neurons, 44

interview methodologies, 34–38

interview questions, 36

J

James, Rick, 18

Janischewsky, Dmitrij, 70

jazz, cannabis and, 13

Jbones, 47, 53, 62, 89

joint, 228

journal, cannabis, 216–222

Just Say No campaign, 18

K

Kaplan, Josh, 33, 45, 49, 59

Karan, Mark, 180–185

Kerouac, Jack, 16

kief, 228

Kleon, Austin, 2

Kosher Kush, 68

L

Lamarck, Jean-Baptiste, 70

landrace strains, 75, 228

legalization of cannabis, 4, 220

limonene, 68

linalool, 68

Linnaeus, Carl, 70

M

MAC, 68

mainstream use, 18

Malysa, Dariusz, 48, 51, 61

Mandelaveitia, Carlos, 117–123

Marcus, Edward, 52, 57, 63

Marihuana Tax Act of 1937, 15

market, cannabis, 85–87

Marley, Bob, 18

Marras, Michael, 112–116

Marx, Groucho, 15

McDowell, Mark, 198–202

McQueen, Steve, 15

medical use, origins of, 10

Mendoza, Kael, 57, 175–179

metabolic enzymes, 41

Mezzrow, Mezz, 13

microdosing, 54, 228

Mitchum, Robert, 15

Monroe, Marilyn, 15

moonrocks, 228

Moreau, Jacques Joseph, 12

music, cannabis and, 13, 18

musicians, 100–106, 124–128, 152–156, 157–163, 169–174, 180–185

myrcene, 69

N

National Institute on Drug Abuse, 4

nausea suppression, 42, 67

Nelson, Willie, 19

neurotransmitters, 42

Nicholson, Jack, 16

NIDA, 4

Nixon, Richard, 18

O

O'Riley, Christopher, 124–128

OG Kush, 69

OutKast, 18

outward-in mentality, 59–60

P

pain relief, 42

Patel, Sanjay, 46, 51

performers, 186–190

photo credits, 229

photographers, 186–190, 203–212

physiological response, 54

pinene, 69

Poehler, Robert, 191–197

Pollock, Anna, 62, 136–141

prohibition of cannabis, 15

prompts, 221–222

propaganda, cannabis and, 14, 18, 19

psychotropic, 228

psychoactive properties of pot, 66

Purple Hindu Kush, 68

Q

qualitative research, 33–38

R

racism, cannabis and, 14, 18

Reagan, Nancy, 18

Reagan, Ronald, 18

references, 230–232

regulations, research, 4–6

religion, cannabis and, 10

Remote Associates Test (RAT), 30

research, cannabis, 4–8, 30–34

    biases, 37

    early documentation, 13

    interviews, 7

    Moreau, Jacques Joseph, 12

    scientific, 4–6, 30–34

    top-down approach, 54–55

response to cannabis, 54

Rivera, Diego, 19

Rogan, Seth, 19

ruderalis, 71

Ruger, Nelson, cover, 142–148

S

Sagan, Carl, 19

salience network, 25

sativa vs indica, 70–74

    classification, 78, 86

sativa, 73

scientific research, barriers to, 4–6

sculptors, 112–116

seizures, treatment of, 67

self-awareness, 24

self-consciousness, 24

Shore, Garrett, 129–135

Smith, Trisha, 46, 62, 89

smoking, 87

Snoop Dogg, 18

Sour Diesel, 69

spliff, 228

sploof, 228

steamroller, 228

stigmas, 81

strains

    classification, 78, 86

    common names, 68–69

    genetics, 76–78

    naming, 77

stress, cannabis and, 45

sugar leaves, 81

T

taproot, 80

tasting notes, 221–222

Taylor, Elizabeth, 15

terpenes, 68–69

tetrahydrocannabinol, see THC

THC, 40, 66, 228

    delta-8 vs delta-9, 66

    percentage, 4

theatre, 191–197

Thompson, Hunter S., 19

top-down approach, 54–55

Tosh, Peter, 18

trichomes, 81, 228

trimming, 84

Tupac, 18

U

Uncle Sexy, 46, 53, 56, 62, 90

US cannabis farm, 4

user experience, 87–92, 214–222

    tracking, 219–220

V

Valdez, Daniela, 92, 107–111

vaping, 87

vaporizer, 228

vegetative stage, 82

Villamin, Kay, 203–212

visual artists, 112–116, 129–135, 136–141, 142–148, 157–163, 164–168, 186–190, 198–202

volcano, 228

W

War on Drugs, 18

wax, 228

Wedding Cake, 68

Weil, Andrew, 34

White Widow, 69

Williams, Kenton, 152–156

Williams, Laurel, 48, 52, 56, 61, 89

Wingfield Jr., Gary, 53, 57, 63

Wright, Cassius, 58, 92

writers, 95–99, 107–111, 149–151

Wu-Tang Clan, 18

Wu, Bruno, 48, 52, 57, 90, 92